Living Sexuality
Issues for Nursing and Health

Edited by
Christine Webb BA, MSc, PhD, RGN, RSCN, RNT
Professor of Nursing, University of Manchester
with nine contributors

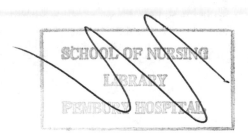

SCUTARI PRESS
London

© Scutari Press 1994

A division of Scutari Projects, the publishing company of the Royal College of Nursing.

First published 1994

British Library Cataloguing in Publication Data

Webb, Christine
  Living Sexuality
  I. Title
  306.7

  ISBN 1–873853–01–7
Typeset by J&L Composition, Filey, North Yorkshire
Printed by Bell and Bain Ltd, Glasgow.

Living Sexuality

Contents

Foreword

My first book on this topic – *Sexuality, Nursing and Health* – was published in 1985. When the publishers asked me to consider a second edition, I was reluctant both because things have moved on a great deal in relation to nursing interest in sexuality, but also because in other ways things have not changed.

In the first book I discussed theories of sexuality, its relationship to the history of nursing, and how we could bring issues of sexuality into nursing care. I presented and critiqued the classic literature on biological, psychological and sociological explanations of sexuality and gender differences. Now, almost a decade later, this work is still largely valid because those studies have remained the foundations of debates about sexuality. Thus, I did not feel that I could update these parts of the original book.

In another way, nurses' knowledge and practice in relation to sexuality and nursing care have made great strides. I would like to think that this is partly as a result of my earlier book, which was the first of its kind for nurses on this side of the Atlantic. Since then Jan Savage has published *Nurses, Gender and Sexuality*, and Jean Glover has written *Human Sexuality in Nursing Care*. Nurses have responded to all these books by becoming aware that sexuality has been a neglected area of practice in relation both to patients and nurses themselves. Evidence for this claim is the fact that a CINAHL computer search for 1992 – the last complete year for which data are available – shows that 125 articles were published on the topic, whereas the list for 1986 includes only 65 titles.

Instead of a second edition, then, I had the idea of producing a book which took for granted this burgeoning interest in sexuality in relation to nursing by focusing on particular examples bringing together research on sexuality and nursing practice. I asked a group of specialists for whom sexuality was an important focus of their research and practice to contribute a chapter to a new book, and to draw explicit links between their work and nursing care.

This volume is the result of our endeavours and I hope readers will find that it extends their thinking and gives pointers to developing nursing practice in relation to sexuality, nursing and care.

References

Glover J (1985) *Human Sexuality in Nursing Care*. London: Croom Helm.
Savage J (1987) *Nurses, Gender and Sexuality*. London: Heinemann.
Webb C (1985) *Sexuality, Nursing and Health*. Chichester: J. Wiley.

Acknowledgements

Thanks go to Jane Hough, who helped with word processing, and struggled womanfully with the task of converting discs from one word processing package to another – demonstrating once again that technology makes life more complicated rather than easier for women. I am grateful too for Kath Foley's help with reviewing the literature for Chapter 10.

Some of the material from Chapter 10 originally appeared in articles in the *Journal of Advanced Nursing* and *Advances in Health and Nursing Care*. I am grateful to the editors of these journals for permission to use this material.

Notes on Contributors

Mary Black graduated in Sociology from the universities of York and Leeds in the early 1970s. After working at the Equal Opportunities Commission, managing research on women's employment issues, she carried out a research project on the Tameside Nursing Development Unit and obtained an MSc from the University of Manchester. She now works at the Centre for Primary Care Research at the University of Manchester.

Jean Faugier is Senior Lecturer at the University of Manchester Community Nursing Professional Unit. She trained as a psychiatric nurse and later as a psychotherapist. She has undertaken a number of research projects investigating HIV and drug misuse, the most recent being a study for the Department of Health on drug-using prostitutes and their risk behaviour. She is currently undertaking a secondment to the Nursing Division of the Department of Health, and is a member of the Home Office Advisory Council on the Misuse of Drugs.

Kath Ferguson trained as a psychiatric nurse in 1984, after a brief period of experience in general nursing. She has worked both in hospital and community settings, specialising in acute care and drug dependency. From 1987–1990 she taught social sciences to health professionals at Salford College of Technology, and currently works as a lecturer in nursing (mental health) at the University of Manchester.

Liz Jones took a BSc in Nursing at Leeds Polytechnic and then moved to London where, after several staff nurse posts, she joined the Royal Marsden Hospital and stayed until 1988 – latterly as a tutor to the oncology nursing courses. In 1983–1984 she took an MSc in Nursing Education at the University of Edinburgh. In 1991 she received funding from the Cancer Relief Macmillan Fund which enabled her to undertake an ethnography of the experiences of young men with testicular cancer. She was appointed to a Macmillan Lectureship in the School of Nursing Studies at the University of Manchester in 1993.

Vina Mayor is Senior Lecturer in Nursing Studies at the University of Hertfordshire. She is a Kenyan Asian (Hindu–Punjabi). Her research interests are health visiting practice; race and health; and gender, race and career development. She is currently undertaking part-time PhD studies, investigating the career patterns of black nurses.

Liz Meerabeau was Head of the School of Advanced Nursing at the North East Surrey College of Technology (NESCOT), in Surrey at the time of writing her chapter. After working as a health visitor for six years, she spent twelve years in various posts in nursing and health visiting education, during which time she completed her PhD looking at the experiences of couples undergoing fertility investigations. Her other interests include the sociology of the emotions, and the 'new public management' in the public sector (sparked by a recent MBA course). She has recently become a research officer at the Department of Health.

Michael Morgan was born in Belfast in 1956. He was educated initially by the Christian Brothers, before gaining degrees in Social Sciences, first at the Northern Ireland Polytechnic (as it then was) and latterly at Queen's University Belfast. Michael was diagnosed as having Friedreich's ataxia in childhood, and has been a wheelchair-user since shortly after his twenty-first birthday. He currently works as a freelance journalist, contributing to a wide variety of local, national and British publications, and is also editor of *Euro-ataxia*, journal of the European Federation of Hereditary Ataxias, of which he is a co-founder.

David Shaw is Principal Lecturer in the Faculty of Health Studies at Buckinghamshire College, which is part of Brunel University. He has a clinical background in cardiac nursing but has worked in nursing education since 1978. In his present post he teaches psychology and health studies on a variety of nursing and health and welfare courses and acts as Course Leader to the Project 2000 course. He has, over the years, developed a keen interest in the psychosocial aspects of coronary heart disease and considers this to be his specialism. In his 'spare' time he engages in post-coronary and bereavement counselling.

Pat Turton is a lecturer in nursing at the University of Manchester, and her background is in anthropology and district nursing. From 1989 to 1993 she was seconded to North Manchester District Health Authority as Nurse Specialist for HIV/AIDS patients in the community. During the secondment she carried out an action research project to establish what changes in service provision would enable people with HIV-related illness to be cared for at home, and to bring about or facilitate such changes.

Christine Webb is Professor of Nursing at the University of Manchester. After qualifying as a nurse, she took a degree in Sociology and then returned to nursing in several clinical and educational posts. She obtained a PhD for her research on recovery from hysterectomy, and has concentrated on issues of women's health and sexuality in subsequent research and teaching. She has previously published a book on *Sexuality, Nursing and Health*. Her current research interest is the health of women of different marital statuses in old age.

ix

Chapter 1
Living Sexuality
Christine Webb

Introduction

Living sexuality has two meanings in the title of this book. First, it conveys the idea that the issues discussed are living ones, in the sense of being current topics of vital concern. But secondly, it emphasises that the lives of the patients and nurses whose stories feature in the book are very much influenced by their sexuality – they are living their sexuality, often in particularly poignant ways.

Nurses now recognise that sexuality is not just about biological functioning and reproductive behaviour, but that a person's sexuality involves their whole personality and is a pervasive influence on every aspect of life. How we present ourselves to others in our body language and dress gives them messages about our sexuality, and we adopt these styles of presentation as an expression of our self-concept of ourselves as sexual beings. Whether the messages we send are received by others in the way we intend is not so straightforward, but the influence of sexuality in our lives is nevertheless far-reaching. As Susan Poorman puts it,

> Sexuality is interwoven with every aspect of human existence . . . Humans express and live their sexuality in their daily lives . . . [in] the way we relate to others, our friends, our family, and our work. It is evident in what we believe, how we behave, and the way we look.
>
> (Poorman 1988, 1)

Changing Lives

Some aspects of sexuality are changing perhaps more rapidly within our lifetimes than in any other age. *Social Trends*, the government statistical summary for 1993, shows this changing picture in a striking way (Central

Statistical Office 1993). It reveals that in 1961 11 per cent of households consisted of one person only, but by 1991 this had increased to 27 per cent. Lone parents with dependent children formed 8 per cent of families in 1972, but by 1991 this had risen to 18 per cent. Over the past 20 years, lone mothers with dependent children have risen from 7 to 17 per cent of families, while lone fathers and their children remained constant at 1 per cent. The percentage of families consisting of a married couple and their dependent children fell from 92 per cent in 1972 to 83 per cent in 1991. Thus, fewer people now live in the traditional nuclear family, and conversely more single parent families exist.

These changes can be understood by looking at the *Social Trends* figures for divorce and reproductive behaviour. Whereas in 1961 the divorce rate in England and Wales was 2.1 per thousand married people, in 1990 it was 12.9. The divorce rate has increased for marriages of up to 4 years' duration, so dissolution is much more common in the early years of marriage.

Perhaps the most striking statistics are those for conceptions and births outside marriage. In 1971 3.5 per cent of births outside marriage were registered in the joint names of both parents, while in 1990 this had risen to 17.6 per cent, showing a five-fold rise in the numbers deciding not to legalise their partnership despite giving birth to a child. The numbers of women registering a birth solely in their own names increased from 4.1 per cent to 6.2 per cent over the same 20-year period. Thus, fewer couples feel the need for a legally binding marriage contract, and more women are choosing to bring up children alone.

Abortion statistics also reveal profound changes over the last two decades. In 1971 just over 44,000 single women had abortions, but in 1991 this figure had risen to 118,000. The comparative figures for married women were 41,500 and 39,200, showing a slight decrease. Abortions in women under 16 years of age decreased by a half, while those for women over 45 increased seven-fold.

These changes in some of the ways in which people express their sexuality are clearly related to changes in divorce and abortion laws, as well as changes in contraceptive technology and use and in techniques for detecting fetal abnormalities which are particularly likely to occur in older women.

Changing Families

Social and demographic changes in the 20th century affect how people's lives develop in different ways from previously (O'Rand and Henretta 1982). People are marrying later and therefore fertility rates have declined. Childbearing either takes place early or is postponed for career reasons as two-worker families become the norm rather than the exception. Divorce and remarriage have increased and divorce has replaced widowhood as a cause of single parent families, the overwhelming majority of which are headed by women, as we have seen.

In addition, people are now living much longer, and women now live half of their lives after childrearing is complete. Therefore, to see female life cycles in terms of reproduction is inappropriate. Childcare is being replaced by obligations to support older parents, and middle-aged people are subject to 'intergenerational squeeze' (O'Rand and Henretta 1982) between the pressures of caring for both children and parents. Far from suffering a mid-life crisis and depression due to the 'empty nest syndrome', some research suggests that women's emotional wellbeing increases when children leave home, and that depression is greater in women whose children remain at home after their expected departure time (Lowenthal and Chiriboga 1972, Barnett and Baruch 1978).

Those who had their own children at a very young age are now grandparents by mid-life and can expect to become great-grandparents. Changing patterns of childrearing, divorce and remarriage may particulary affect people in mid-life (Sprey and Mathews 1982). Families today may consist of a man or woman's own children and those of their second marriage partner brought from the first marriage. The family may also be widened to include all the grandparents of these step-grandchildren, and thus the number of in-laws in the family increases. One resulting problem to which we have not yet developed a solution is what to call these 'relations'.

Teenage pregnancy may also mean that mid-life grandparents take over financial and childcare responsibilities for a grandchild at a time when they were expecting to be free from parental responsibilities, or young people with children may ask a grandmother in her mid-40s to look after children while they work, leading to conflict for her because she wants to return to employment after bringing up her own children.

Complex transitions, therefore, may coincide for all family members, as parents reach mid-life and children grow up. Divorce and remarriage may affect both generations, and the strains for women at mid-life may be greater than for men because of their multiple role responsibilities as wives, mothers and workers. However, Wilsnack and Cheloha (1987), in a study of problem drinking, found that multiple roles did not contribute to mid-life stress. On the contrary, they provided women with self-esteem and social support, as well as little time for drinking!

That employment enhances women's health and protects them against stress is a finding of much research (Madans and Verbrugge 1983), although it may be that part-time work outside the home leads to a better balance between 'role enhancement' and 'role overload' (Bartley, Popay and Plewis 1992). Paid work reduces women's sense of isolation, builds their self-esteem and gives them a higher sense of 'prestige' (Rosenfeld 1989). For women in professional and managerial jobs, however, mental and physical health may be put at risk if they work and compete under pressure. The 'executive stress' traditionally associated with men may be a cost paid by women entering the labour force at this level.

Nurses' enhanced self-esteem and job satisfaction when working in a nursing development unit that allows them to feel that they are making a positive contribution to the care of their elderly patients is discussed by Mary Black in Chapter 11.

Marriage itself is not necessarily beneficial to women's self-esteem – it is the emotional quality of the marital relationship that is more important for them (Gove, Hughes and Style 1983). For men, marriage itself is more important because they gain material and emotional services carried out for them by their wives. Men remarry more quickly after divorce because they feel unable to cope without these services, usually having fewer social ties to their children and losing their principal confidante. Women are likely to retain closer contact with the children and to have a wider range of confidantes.

Changes in family life, therefore, have far-reaching effects on all family members, whether they are parents who have their children when they themselves are very young or whether they postpone having children until their careers are established. The later generation, too, is profoundly affected by their children's life choices as well as their own, in the spheres of marital relationships, work and caring for younger or older family members.

These changes mean that we are living our sexuality – both in reproductive and social senses – very differently from the previous generations. Therefore we do not have ready-made ways of dealing with these transitions and we have to work these out as we go along. This applies just as much to changing female and male roles at home and work as to what to call new people who suddenly become part of our families as a result of divorce and remarriage and how to relate to them.

Issues of sexuality and mental health are taken up by Kath Ferguson in Chapter 7, where she considers concerns both for clients and for nurses themselves. Her chapter discusses the variations in mental health problems according to gender, and discusses some possible explanations of this, highlighting the challenges raised for nursing practice.

New Women?

'Post-feminism' is a term used to describe the supposedly more fair and equal society that now exists in the West following the 'women's liberation move-ment' of the 1970s and 1980s. Since the Sex Discrimination Act came into effect in 1976, so the thinking goes, there is no longer any need to be divisive. Women and men are living and working together on a more equal basis than ever before; and 'new men' are more in touch with their feelings, share housework more equally, and increasingly play a part in bringing up their children.

On the other hand, there are claims that any advances in women's position as a result of the women's liberation movement are now leading to a 'backlash' (Faludi 1991) or a 'war against women' (French 1992). Even leaving aside the fact that any gains for women have taken place largely in western societies, there is much dispute about the reality of these gains.

Housework and childcare are still very much a woman's province. Figures from the Department of Employment in 1984 show that, even when the woman in a family is working full-time, her male partner contributes little to these tasks (OPCS 1984). Fifty-four per cent of women working full-time said that they did all or most of the housework, and only 44 per cent said there was equal sharing. Twenty-nine per cent of full-time women workers and 44 per cent of part-timers said they did most or all of the childcare. However, when men were asked how much they contributed they always claimed to be doing more than their wives described. It also seems that men's and women's contributions differ in quality as well as quantity. In the same study, researchers wrote that:

> Wives are more likely to be involved in the routine basic care such as feeding, dressing, washing and so on, while husbands spent time playing with the children or taking them out.
>
> (OPCS 1984)

The theory–practice gap seems to apply not only to nursing! Financial reasons were given by women as their main reason for working in a survey by Martin and Roberts (OPCS 1984). Similarly, the 50 per cent of married women who were economically active in 1980 (General Household Survey 1982) worked to buy basic essentials for their families, not for luxuries or 'extras'. However, women's weekly earnings were only 70.9 per cent of men's earnings in 1992 (Equal Opportunities Commission 1992).

Women are still concentrated in office work, service industries and manufacturing. Paradoxically, while men's employment has been declining, opportunities for women have increased. However, they have increased in the service industries and in part-time work in fields such as assembly work in the computer industries. Even in professional work where women formerly worked in greater numbers, de-skilling and loss of status are occurring as more auxiliaries are being brought into nursing, social work and similar occupations (Beechey and Whitelegg 1986).

For men, jobs formerly based on physical prowess have either been replaced by computerised technology or have disappeared with economic recession. This has taken its toll on men's mental health and self-esteem (Whelan, Hannan and Creighton 1991) and unemployed men resent the fact that their wives have taken over their traditional breadwinner role (Coote and Campbell 1987).

Clearly, changes in our working lives have great implications for the way we live our sexuality, just as family changes do. And, of course, the two cannot be separated. Work-related stress and unemployment will lead to financial difficulties that in turn will rebound on relationships (Whelan 1993).

The backlash or war against women takes the form, according to French (1992) and Faludi (1991), of a growth of 'new right' calls for a return to traditional family values, with claims that children suffer because their mothers go out to work, and also with continued discrimination against women in all spheres of life. Nurseries are closing, job conditions are deteriorating, and 'care in the community' means that women will be forced to shoulder even more of the burden of caring for the sick and older people (Segal 1987).

At the other end of the spectrum, Lynne Segal (1987) believes that the 'separateness' and oppositional position of the 1970s women's movement is now out of place. She thinks that the time is now ripe to work 'for a future which rejects most of the social distinctions we now draw between women and men'. Similarly Cynthia Cockburn believes that:

> All the true diversity that people are capable of experiencing and expressing, of needing in their sexual, domestic and working lives and of contributing to society, is repressed by gender . . . The good qualities deemed masculine – courage, strength and skill, for instance – and the good qualities seen as feminine – tenderness, the ability to feel and express feelings – should be the qualities available to all . . . regardless of the sex of the person.
>
> (Cockburn 1985, 252)

The quotation uses the word 'gender' instead of 'sex', and this seems to be an increasing trend which is more than simply a use of different words. For example, college courses are now more likely to be called 'Gender Studies' than 'Women's Studies', and bookshops and libraries have often changed the labels on their shelves in the same way. This change of words reflects different ways of thinking of the kind Segal and Cockburn are writing about. The changed terminology reveals a belief that it is more important to focus on understanding both women and men and how we can bring about social changes that will benefit everyone than to focus exclusively on difference and opposition.

Debate rages, then, about whether changes in women's lives are real, or only surface changes which disguise the fact that social life carries on much as before as far as sexuality is concerned. But where are the men in all this debate?

New Men?

The 1980s and 1990s have seen the burgeoning of interest in a phenomenon called the 'new man'. The new man is sensitive and caring, emotionally open, wears softer and more colourful clothes, and shares equally in bringing up his children and running the home.

The discovery of this new expression of masculinity has been the subject of a number of books, and authors make links between women's struggles for greater equality, the development of women's studies courses and the gay movement. In *Discovering Men*, Morgan (1992) writes that 'the search for men . . . has been initiated by women', and he talks of men and 'masculinities' because he believes that it is not appropriate to see all men as behaving in the same way. He is critical of the negative aspects of traditional masculinity and wants to explore, analyse and change the use of violence by men, for example. But he also thinks that it is important to appreciate 'the positive features of men's lives, and especially the variety of men's lived experiences'.

'Unwrapping masculinity' is the task of Chapman and Rutherford's book *Male Order* (Chapman and Rutherford 1988). They consider that 'the forward march of men' towards different kinds of behaviour has been halted – or at least impeded – by social and economic changes, including the 'new right' political moves to re-assert male authority. Evidence of this is seen in both calls for a return to Victorian values and in the anti-gay (or homophobic) stance of the infamous 'clause 28' of the Local Government and Finance Bill and newspapers such as the *Star* and *Sun*. Chapman and Rutherford's book is about

> the necessity for men to redefine masculinity, to imagine and produce new forms of sexual and erotic expression, to produce a masculinity whose desire is no longer dependent on oppression, no longer policed by homophobia, and one that no longer resorts to violence and misogyny to maintain its sense of coherence.
>
> (Chapman and Rutherford 1988, 18)

Chapman and Rutherford acknowledge that their project to achieve a more democratic and emancipated society in the next century 'will require a long journey', and many other commentators agree with them. Polly Toynbee wrote in the *Guardian* in 1987 that

> The New Man is not here, and it does not seem likely that we shall see him in our lifetime, nor in our children's.

In their book '*Reassessing Fatherhood: New Observations on Fathers and the Modern Family*, Lewis and O'Brien (1987) also have difficulty locating evidence about the reality of a new paternal role, indeed, men's contribution to work in the home is increasing at about 24 seconds in every 10 years. While 98 per cent of men attend the births of their babies, the amount of nappy-changing and baby-bathing they do leads the authors to conclude that

> It has been impossible to define any essential role for fathers, other than that of a supportive family member and friend . . .

and that there is no evidence 'of the vital role model that fathers provide for sons'. The problem is that fathers simply do not know how to make the time they spend with their children 'quality time'.

Men are increasingly seeking custody of their children after divorce but Phillips (1992) is sceptical about whether awarding custody to fathers is the right decision. Men – whether they have custody or only access rights – do spend more time with their children after divorce, but this largely reflects how little time they spent with them beforehand. There is also evidence that father residence is slightly worse for (children of) both sexes, although boys seem to be pretty much the same with either parent, and girls show some negative effects of living with fathers.

Phillips' conclusion is that what is important for children is people who can form warm and close relationships with them, and that most children will be happier with the parent who spent most time with them before the divorce took place.

Violence and abuse within the family have also leapt to our attention in recent years. This violence is overwhelmingly perpetrated by men against women and children, and this is because 'the boundaries of correct behaviour are just not the same for men and women', according to researchers at Bradford University (Utley 1993). Men questioned in the study saw violence as meaning physical attacks resulting in injuries, but did not think that pushing, physical restraint or throwing women about counted as violence, nor did psychological nor emotional violence. Furthermore, they did not see forced sex as constituting violence. The researchers conclude that stopping men's violence will entail changing definitions of what is socially acceptable and making this a public policy campaign.

So far, then, it seems that the 'new man' is a rare and endangered species and that bringing about changes in attitudes and behaviour will be a very long haul indeed.

Living Longer

Reproductive matters such as contraception and abortion were main campaigning issues in the 1970s and 1980s, but as women who took up these struggles themselves have grown older their attention has moved on to new issues. Germaine Greer (1991) has written about older women's increasing interest in the menopause, and in what she and others see as the largely male medical profession's continued attempt to control women's health and turn health issues into pathological conditions needing treatment.

The only symptoms which can definitely be linked with the menopause are hot flushes and sweating (Greene 1980), and part of the problem is that the normal menopause has received little attention (Voda and George 1986). This may be related to the fact that the 'experts' on the subject have been mainly men – doctors or psychologists – who are trained to deal with abnormalities and who have never had similar experiences themselves. As Kahana and Kahana (1982, 146) say:

One explanation for this may be that society's labelling of menopause as a highly stressful event is based on stereotyped notions offered by persons who have not experienced this event. Middle aged women are far more likely to provide positive evaluations of middle age changes than are persons in younger age groups. The majority of middle-aged women attribute little discontinuity in their lives to the climacterium and . . . women rate menopause as requiring little adjustment when compared with other life events.

While some doctors and women hail hormone replacement treatment (HRT) as the answer, others are worried about several aspects of this approach. They fear the side-effects and possible carcinogenic influence of HRT, and prefer to deal with the change as part of life's normal transitions. Taking care of one's own health by having a healthy diet and exercise, not over-indulging in alcohol and cigarette-smoking, and taking time for oneself are seen as more positive choices than HRT and other medications because they have no side-effects and give women a feeling of control over their own lives (Greer 1991).

Asian women's experiences of the menopause are discussed by Vina Mayor in Chapter 8. She set up a project to give information to a group of women living in an inner city where they felt that health professionals were not always sensitive to their needs. They wanted information about the menopause, and told Vina Mayor about their own cultural beliefs and attitudes. This chapter graphically brings home the necessity for health workers to try to understand and respect the varying understandings and beliefs of their client groups and their need for health-related information and advice.

Ageing, too, is increasingly being taken up as an issue by women who were previously concerned about reproductive issues, and Barbara Macdonald (Macdonald and Rich 1984) has written poignantly of her sadness and anger at being discriminated against by other women on the grounds of her age. Acknowledgement that ageing is a growing concern for women also comes from academic research. The common belief that retirement is an important and stressful life event for men but not for women is countered by research showing that post-retirement adjustment can be more difficult for women. They have to face not only the loss of their job, with its financial and esteem-building rewards, and fewer social contacts, but are usually obliged to continue with a housework role and possibly to take care of ageing relatives or spouses. For a woman who was not employed previously, the retirement of her partner forces them together for much more of the time than before, and she loses part of the independence she had when alone in the home for a large part of the day. Because they tend to live longer than men, women are also more likely to undergo the stress of widowhood and other bereavements (Reinharz 1986, Russell 1987).

Women who have chosen not to marry are no less likely than those who have married to be vulnerable and to experience difficulties as they grow older, as Macdonald and Rich (1984) report. Their support networks are likely to be smaller, their financial position more precarious and their long-fought-for independence threatened. These and other aspects of the life and health of elderly, never-married women are discussed in Chapter 10 by Christine Webb.

For men, too, the 'retirement syndrome' of loss of status and identity, financial stress and difficulties in filling time may be followed by poor health and premature death following the loss of their principal life activity (Ley 1981). The links between sexuality and ageing should therefore concern us all, both as individuals and as health care workers.

Sexuality and Health

Sexuality and health are closely related, sometimes in obvious and other times in unexpected ways. Coronary heart disease – the leading cause of early death in Britain – is often seen as a male problem, for example. The idea of Type A and Type B personalities is now part of popular health understandings, and the typical coronary patient is usually thought of as a man working under stress in a high pressure, executive-type job. The reality is a mixture of these ideas. Coronary heart disease is more prevalent in the lower social classes than among middle-class workers (Whitehead 1988), and the gap between men and women in mortality has decreased in recent years (Marmot and McDowell 1986). David Shaw takes up these issues in Chapter 9, and shows how an awareness of the complex inter-relationships between gender and heart disease can be used by nurses to offer more appropriate health education and counselling to coronary heart disease patients.

Cancer is another major cause of morbidity and mortality which can have overt as well as less obvious links with sexuality. Nurses have become increasingly aware of the potentially devastating effect of breast cancer on women's mental health, and research has shown that interventions by nurses after surgery can be effective in promoting recovery and in early detection of depressive symptoms (Maguire et al 1980, 1983). Less attention has been given to sexuality-related issues and male cancer. Liz Jones and Christine Webb report on an interview study of young men experiencing testicular cancer in Chapter 3, and discuss how the men underwent a journey through diagnosis and treatments to emerge seeing 'the light at the end of the tunnel'. Masculine self-concept and fertility were concerns for them on the journey, but the quality of their relationships with and support from significant others was also crucial to coping.

No book of this kind today can ignore issues of sexuality, HIV and AIDS. In the early 1980s when AIDS first came to our attention, almost all cases were homosexual men in their late twenties and early thirties. This led to a certain amount of public moralising and panic, and to the coining of the term 'gay plague' by the more sensational section of the media. Soon, however, it became clear that intravenous drug use was another mode of spread to both men and women, and that bisexual people were also at risk (Illman 1993). In 1993 there are thought to be 12 million HIV-positive adults in the world, of whom 40 per cent are women (Panos Institute 1993). The idea that HIV and AIDS predominantly affect young people who then die prematurely is also false. About 1000 older people in the UK are estimated to be HIV positive and the course of AIDs runs faster in older people, with some symptoms being mistakenly diagnosed as Alzheimer's disease (Age Concern 1993).

Jean Faugier writes in Chapter 4 about her research with women prostitutes and their clients in relation to HIV and AIDS, and shows the complexity of people's thinking about sexuality. For example, prostitutes may insist that clients use condoms, but may see this as inappropriate for men with whom they have personal and sexual relationships.

Pat Turton (Chapter 5) considers care at home for people dying of AIDS and their partners and families. She found that gay men were reluctant to use community care services for fear of homophobic attitudes on the part of health care staff, and breaches of confidentiality. This chapter also catalogues the multitudinous effects that AIDS can have for both physical and psychosocial aspects of sexuality for patients themselves, and for informal carers and parents of gay men.

Infertility is another issue in which sexuality and health are clearly closely linked and which has come to the fore in recent years with the development of increasingly technical forms of treatment. Cultural definitions of mother-hood as the principal source of women's fulfilment can lead infertile women to see themselves as failures and to suffer corresponding loss of self-esteem, anxiety and depression (Pfeffer 1987). Once a couple become involved in the long, drawn-out process of tests and treatments, life – particularly for the women – can become a chronic crisis. Each monthly period may be a sign of failure, and sexual relationships degenerate into part of the medical process. Men in such couples may experience 'performance anxiety' too (Murdoch 1990), and years may be wasted as costly and potentially risky treatments are repeatedly unsuccessful.

Liz Meerabeau argues, in Chapter 2, that subfertility is a better term than infertility because it is not usually possible to be so certain about outcomes. She writes about investigations, treatments and their effect on couples, and of the role of nurses in helping both those who eventually succeed in having a baby as well as those who need to come to an adjustment that for them adoption or childlessness is what the future holds. She sees the major issues as supporting people in their uncertainty in planning for their futures.

Sexuality and disability is another area receiving increased attention in the past twenty years, as Michael Morgan discusses in Chapter 6. Morgan believes that this 'marked openness in the discussion of sexual matters . . . has put the problem centre-stage in any overall debate on disability – where, indeed, it belongs'. Relationships and physical aspects of disability are considerations, but perhaps more important are the social exclusion and marginalisation experienced by people with disabilities, and the resulting effects on self-esteem. Full integration of people with disabilities at all levels of society is, in Morgan's view, the only way to end this marginalisation.

These are some issues of living sexuality considered in this book. There are many others we could have included and we have inevitably had to make choices; however, this does not mean that we think these other issues are unimportant. We have tried to cover a broad range of topics and interests important for nurses and nursing. Concerns which are part of everyday life but are not illnesses have been included, as well as conditions requiring treatment and care in hospital and in the community. Both physical and mental health problems are discussed, as well as issues for nursing and for nurses themselves. We hope that the book will contribute to the growing awareness of interlinkages between sexuality, nursing and health and to promoting a greater acceptance of the role of nurses in helping patients and clients.

References

Age Concern (1993) *A Crisis of Silence: HIV, AIDS and Older People*. London: Age Concern.

Barnett R C and Baruch G K (1978) Women in the middle years: a critique of research and theory. *Psychology of Women Quarterly*, **32**, 2, 187–197.

Bartley M, Popay J and Plewis I (1992) Domestic conditions, paid employment and women's experience of ill-health. *Sociology of Health and Illness*, **14**, 2, 313–343.

Beechey V and Whitelegg E (1986) *Women in Britain Today*. Milton Keynes: Open University Press.

Central Statistical Office (1993) *Social Trends 23*. London: HMSO.

Chapman R and Rutherford J (eds) (1988) *Male Order. Unwrapping Masculinity*. London: Lawrence and Wishart.

Cockburn C (1985) *Machinery of Dominance: Women, Men and Technical Know-how*. London: Pluto Press.

Coote A and Campbell B (1987) *Sweet Freedom* (2nd edn). Oxford: Blackwell.

Equal Opportunities Commission (1983) *Eighth Annual Report*. Manchester: EOC.

Equal Opportunities Commission (1992) *New Earnings Survey 1971–92*. Manchester: EOC.

Faludi S (1991) *Backlash. The Undeclared War Against Women*. London: Chatto & Windus.

French M (1992) *The War Against Women*. London: Hamish Hamilton.

General Household Survey (1982) London: HMSO.

Gove W R, Hughes M and Style C B (1983) Does marriage have positive effects on the psychological well-being of the individual? *Journal of Health and Social Behaviour*, **24**, 122–131.

Greene J G (1980) Stress in the Phyllosan years. *New Society*, **54**, 18 December, 944–945.

Greer G (1991) *The Change. Women, Ageing and the Menopause*. London: Hamish Hamilton.

Illman J (1993) AIDS/HIV. History lesson. *Nursing Times*, **89**, 26, 26–29.

Kahana B and Kahana E (1982) Clinical issues of middle age and later life. *Annals of the American Academy of Political and Social Science*, **464**, 140–161.

Lewis C and O'Brien M (eds) (1987) *Reassessing Fatherhood: New Observations on Fathers and the Modern Family*. London: Sage.

Ley P (1981) Psychological aspects of aging. Unpublished paper presented at the Behavioural Medicine Conference, Cumberland College of Health Sciences, Sydney, Australia.

Lowenthal M F and Chiriboga D (1972) Transition to the empty nest: crisis, challenge or relief? *Archives of General Psychiatry*, **26**, 8–14.

Macdonald B and Rich C (1984) *Look Me in the Eye: Old Women, Aging and Ageism*. London: The Women's Press.

Madans J H and Verbrugge L M (1983) Trends in health in American women. Unpublished paper.

Maguire P, Tait A, Brooke M, Thomas C and Sellwood R (1980) Effect of counselling on the psychiatric morbidity associated with mastectomy. *British Medical Journal*, **282**, 1454–1456.

Maguire P, Pentol A, Allen D, Tait A, Brooke M, Thomas C and Sellwood T (1983) The effect of counselling on physical disability and social recovery after mastectomy. *Clinical Oncology*, **9**, 319–324.

Marmot M G and McDowell M E (1986) Mortality decline and widening social inequalities. *Lancet*, **2**, 274–276.

Morgan D (1992) *Discovering Men. Critical Studies on Men and Masculinities 3*. London: Routledge.

Murdoch A (1990) Off the treadmill – leaving an IVF programme behind. In Scutt J A (ed) *The Baby Machine. Reproductive Technology and the Commercialisation of Motherhood*. London: Merlin Press.

Office of Population Censuses and Surveys (1984) *Women and Employment*. London: HMSO.

O'Rand A M and Henretta J C (1982) Women at middle age: developmental transitions. *Annals of the American Academy of Political and Social Science*, **464**, November, 57–64.

Panos Institute (1993) *Aids Media Briefing No. 1*. London: Panos Institute.

Pfeffer N (1987) Artificial insemination, in vitro fertilisation and the stigma of infertility. In Stanworth M (ed) *Reproductive Technologies: Gender, Motherhood and Medicine*. Oxford: Polity Press.

Phillips A (1992) The man as mother. *Guardian*, 23.10.92.

Poorman S G (1988) *Human Sexuality and the Nursing Process*. Norwalk, Connecticut: Appleton & Lange.

Reinharz S (1986) Friends or foes: gerontological and feminist theory. *Women's Studies International Forum*, **9**, 5, 503–514.

Rosenfeld S (1989) The effects of women's employment, personal control and sex differences in mental health. *Journal of Health and Social Behaviour*, **30**, 77–91.

Russell C (1987) Ageing as a feminist issue. *Women's Studies International Forum*, **10**, 2, 125–132.

Segal L (1987) *Is the Future Female? Troubled Thoughts on Contemporary Feminism*. London: Virago.

Sprey J and Mathews S H (1982) Contemporary grandparenthood: a systemic transition. *Annals of the American Academy of Political and Social Science*, **464**, November, 91–103.

Toynbee P (1987) The incredible, shrinking New Man. *Guardian*, 6.4.87.

Utley A (1993) Wife-beaters deny violent behaviour. *The Times Higher Education Supplement*, 2.7.93.

Voda A M and George T (1986) Menopause. *Annual Review of Nursing Research*, **4**, 55–75.

Whelan C T (1993) The role of social support in mediating the psychological consequences of economic stress. *Sociology of Health and Illness*, **15**, 1, 86–101.

Whelan C T, Hannan D F and Creighton S (1991) Unemployment, poverty and psychological distress. The Economic and Social Research Institute, General Research Series Paper No. 150, Dublin.

Whitehead M (1988) *The health divide*. Harmondsworth: Penguin.

Wilsnack R W and Cheloha R (1987) Women's roles and problem drinking across the lifespan. *Social Problems*, **34**, 3, 231–248.

Chapter 2
Fertility and Reproductive Technology
Liz Meerabeau

Introduction

Fertility problems are common in both the US and the UK, and are estimated to affect one in six couples at some stage in their lives (Hull 1985), although this may be an overestimate (Pfeffer and Quick 1988). Generally, a problem is defined if the woman has not conceived after a year of unprotected intercourse. Many readers of this book are likely to have experienced problems themselves, or to have friends with problems. Many nurses will work with subfertile women in various health care settings, such as gynaecology wards; practice nurses may be involved with preparing women for IVF (in vitro fertilisation). Nurses will also encounter involuntarily childless people in other health care settings. It is therefore a topic which concerns all of us.

In this chapter, I will concentrate on the social effects of subfertility; for details of medical treatments, readers are referred to Abdalla, Baber and Studd (1990), Ng et al (1988) and Seibel (1990). I am using the term subfertility rather than infertility, since it is rarely possible to state that someone has no chance of achieving parenthood; the uncertainty this can create will be discussed further below. For clarity, I will refer to couples, while recognising that single women also seek treatment, particularly donor insemination (Heywood, 1991). I will also concentrate mainly on the experience of couples who have either primary subfertility (that is, have never conceived) or those who have conceived, but have not succeeded in producing a live child. Much of the literature concerns these two groups, who are not parents, and it may be that the experience of parenting an only child and being unable to achieve a sibling is quite different. For the social context, I have confined myself to British and American and a small amount of Australian and New Zealand literature, but it is important to bear in mind that the meaning of subfertility will be affected by the meaning of parenthood in a particular society (see, for example, McGilvray 1982, Baluch, Manyande and Aghssa 1993). Several writers have claimed that both the US and the UK are

14

pronatalist societies (Veevers 1979), meaning that there is a pressure on couples, and particularly women, to have children, and that those who do not are seen as deviant and stigmatised (Busfield and Paddon 1977, Baum 1980, Campbell 1985, Woollett 1991).

Despite the variety of lifestyles in the US and UK, most young adults expect that they will become parents, and even the phrase 'family planning' implies that conception is straightforward. Houghton and Houghton (1984) say that the childless are pictured as living sad and bitter lives, surrounded by material objects and pets, whereas Pfeffer (1987a) and Franklin (1990) discuss the way in which the media portray subfertile women as 'obsessed' and 'desperate'.

One of the feminist criticisms of fertility treatment is that it emphasises parenthood as the only successful outcome of treatment, rather than helping couples (particularly women) to develop other life goals (Strickler 1992). The relative privacy of the nuclear family in the UK and US reduces opportunities for the childless to care for other people's children, and Elias (1985) claims that in modern societies we do not easily express emotion, except to pets and young children. Much of the literature on parenthood indicates that the onus of parenting still falls most heavily on the mother (see, for example, Lewis and O'Brien 1987); it is therefore not surprising that women are generally found to be more isolated by subfertility than are men (e.g. Greil, Leitko and Porter 1988), although men may feel more stigmatised by a fertility problem.

The issue of whether fertility treatments should be available in an over-populated world surfaces from time to time, particularly since most problems do not affect physical health. Reproductive technology is one of the few treatments to have been rationed explicitly, and a recent application of the Oregon experiment in the UK found it ranked 701 out of 714 treatments in order of priority (Dixon and Gilbert Welch 1991). This issue may be gaining added piquancy in the NHS, given the current purchaser–provider split. In many areas of the country there are no specialist fertility services. The Warnock Report called for a national survey; although this was never carried out, a survey was commissioned by Frank Dobson, then Shadow Minister of Health (Mathieson 1986), and updated by Harriet Harman (1990). A survey of London has also been carried out (Pfeffer and Quick 1988), and a new national survey is currently being undertaken by the College of Health. The picture obtained is of patchy services; diagnostic services for men are particularly poorly developed.

Ethical and Legal Issues

Since subfertility is not simply about a body dysfunction, but has profound effects upon the lives of many people affected, and also involves responsibilities to potential unborn children, it is understandable that treatments have often been controversial. Many feminists (e.g. Corea 1985) consider that reproductive technologies remove women's control over their own bodies. Pfeffer (1987b) has charted the debate about one of the earliest treatments, artificial insemination by donor. This has been available since the 1930s, but as recently as 1988 only 50 per cent of the public thought it should be legal (Harding 1988). More recently, the technique of IVF has caused controversy, resulting in the Warnock Enquiry (1984) and Enoch Powell's unsuccessful Unborn Child (Protection) Bill in 1985. The Warnock Report led to the establishment of the Interim Licensing Authority and the Human Fertilisation and Embryology Act in 1990. Certain treatments are now licensed, namely those involving gamete donation and IVF, since it involves embryos. However, other fairly technical treatments, such as GIFT (gamete intrafallopian transfer) are not regulated, because they do not involve donated gametes. New techniques for men include micro-epididymal sperm aspiration and SUZI, or subzonal insemination (under the zona pellucida of the ovum), which was legalised in the UK in 1991.

There are some concerns that many of these treatments are offered in the private sector, and that the low success rates of the smaller clinics may not be made clear to patients (Montague 1991). There are also risks involved in ovarian hyperstimulation, both for women undergoing IVF and those donating eggs. The first annual report of the Human Fertilisation and Embryology Authority (1992) gave the best success rate as only 14 'take home' babies per 100 treatment cycles of IVF, and some centres have only two conceptions per 100 cycles. There have been suggestions that a 'league table' should be published, although Entwistle (1992) thinks this could lead to the neglect of other indicators, such as the quality of support offered.

It is also important to remember that despite the emphasis given to 'high tech' treatments both by sociologists (McNeil et al 1990, Stacey 1992) and in the press, only a minority of couples undergo them; Montague (1991) estimates less than 3 per cent. The majority have treatments such as hormone therapy. Whereas feminists have feared that women will be forced to have these treatments, others (e.g. Thomas and Heberton 1991) claim that the HFEA's requirement that patients be screened for their suitability to parent will disqualify some women.

The Experience of Subfertility

There have been many studies of the experience of subfertility from a psychological perspective (Humphrey 1975, Allison 1979, Cooper 1979, Feuer 1983). There are also many self-help books written by doctors (see, for example, Winston 1986), or by people who have themselves undergone treatment (Houghton and Houghton 1977, Pfeffer and Woollett 1983). Common themes include the time-consuming nature of treatment, the distress of menstruation and the embarrassment caused by some of the tests, particularly the postcoital test. There have been several sociological studies, for example by Snowden, Mitchell and Snowden (1983) and Snowden and Snowden (1984) of AID (artificial insemination by donor). Owens' (1986) study of 30 Welsh working-class couples explores issues such as conformity and the pressure to parent, and couples' self-concept not as childless, but as prospective parents. Recent American studies include Olshansky's (1987) work with 15 couples, which refers to taking on the identity of subfertility. Sandelowski and Pollock (1986) identify three themes, also found in my own study: the experience of uncertainty and ambiguity, the awareness of time passing, and feelings of being different. One problem with all the studies to date, my own included, is that they are taken from a skewed sample, and some tend to make generalisations which are not really warranted. We have little or no data on people who cannot conceive but who do not seek treatment, since subjects are generally recruited via clinics; demographic data from the US National Survey of Family Growth indicate that there are differences between users and non-users of services (Hirsch and Mosher 1987). Owens tried to interview the patients in a GP practice to ascertain the incidence of involuntary childlessness, but access was refused by the GPs on the grounds of invasion of privacy. Several of the US studies are particularly skewed, since they have recruited from Resolve, the US self-help group, whose membership is estimated to represent only one in 8000 subfertile people. This may be partly why the people in these studies, unlike the British studies to date, seem to be active health care 'consumers' who are very well informed about tests and treatments.

My own study was carried out in the early 1980s (1983–1984) and involved observation in three NHS clinics, plus in-depth taped interviews, usually of two to three hours, with 41 couples and nine women, at various stages of treatment (mean 29 months, range 2 weeks to 10 years). The mean ages were 30 for the women and 32 for the men; working-class couples were under-represented. At least one person in each couple was British, and none had a live child of their marriage, or was caring for young children from a previous marriage. One-third of the women had been pregnant. In 17 couples the woman had a fertility problem; in five couples, the man; in 14, both; and in 14, neither had a problem diagnosed. They were, with three exceptions, interviewed in their own homes. There are disadvantages in interviewing as a couple, since there may be a tendency to present a united front, but the advantage was that it gave some insight into their relationship (Allan 1980). All three clinics observed were either part of a teaching hospital or linked to one, and all three had specialist staff, although most combined subfertility work with gynaecology or urology. None had a fully coordinated service in which specialist help was available for male fertility problems, and they had to refer clients to another centre. IVF was offered within one of the hospitals, although by a different consultant. The range of tests and treatment offered was mainly for ovulatory problems and cervical mucus problems, for which treatment has not changed greatly since my study was carried out.

Men's Participation

Gender differences in the experience of subfertility have been referred to, although emphasis is put on treating the couple. In practice, however, the man may play a peripheral role (Greil et al 1988, Meerabeau 1991). In my study, all but two men had attended at least one clinic appointment, and most were pleased just to be invited into the consultation; those who had greater expectations were disappointed. Of the 19 men with a low sperm count, nine did not think it was a problem, and as indicated above the range of tests and treatment for men is limited. Since most fertility clinics are attached to gynaecology departments, it is easy to see subfertility as a 'women's problem'. Also, as the relationship was not discussed in the clinic, potential conflict between the couple could not be explored (Pfeffer and Woollett 1983).

Emotional Neutrality

One striking finding of mine which is also discussed elsewhere (Hunt and Meerabeau 1993) was the emotional neutrality of the clinics, which echoed that found by Strong (1979) in his study of Scottish paediatric clinics, and which he called the 'bureaucratic format'. The medical literature on subfertility, like that on childhood handicap, refers to guilt and distress, but the subject was never broached in the clinic and when patients did become upset they tried hard to retain their composure. As Strong (1979, 142) states, their tears were their own affair; there might be a pause while they recovered, but sorrow did not become a topic of conversation. I will return to this point in discussing nursing interventions. My interview data indicated that people did not expect the doctors to spend time in discussion; they were described as 'nice but brisk' or 'business-like'. There were no in-depth assessments of why people wanted children, although the HFEA recommends that this should be done more diligently. Strong identified a source of underlying tension in the clinics, which was never really addressed since patients did not wish to seem critical; most people have high expectations of modern medicine, and failure can be seen as failure of the individual doctor. Blame can hang unspoken like a cloud over the consultation, and no remedy is offered for painful feelings other than the solution of the physical problem which has prompted them.

Sexuality and Embarrassment

A further striking finding in my own study was that the professional literature emphasises that the doctor should discuss sexual technique, but this was not done in the consultations I observed. Several studies have discussed the gynaecological examination (Emerson 1970a, b, Henslin and Biggs 1971) and the problem that the genitals are not just like any other part of the body, particularly if the doctor is of the opposite sex. The doctor must maintain a balance between 'the insult of sexual familiarity' and 'the insult of unacknowledged identity' (Emerson 1970b, 85), and the (female) patient must be neither too coy, nor immodest (Goffman 1974). In their encounters with their patients, male gynaecologists may be aided by cultural definitions of women as lacking strong sexual feeling (Scully and Bart 1973). For the man, however, sexuality is linked to performance (Lawler 1991); even the routine male test is not a purely medical act, since it involves masturbation, and is disallowed by some religions even for obtaining a sperm sample. Some of my data obtained from conferences and other sources seem to indicate that male sexuality is rather 'jokey' and/or embarrassing in a way that women's is not, for example the subdued titter when a urologist described to a self-help group how he asked a staff nurse to feel a testicular prosthesis to see whether it felt life-like, amusement about 'splashing his bits with cold water' and wearing boxer shorts as a treatment for oligospermia. Paul, one of my interviewees, commented

I think there's a bit of smoking behind the boys' lav sort of mentality about it, it's all a bit of a laugh, yeah, I think there's a flippant approach. I mean half of it is nervous, isn't it, there for the grace sort of thing . . .

There was not, therefore, any great discussion about either emotional or sexual matters in the clinics, and the couple's relationship was not explored.

Knowledge of Causes and Treatments

A linked finding was that the people interviewed did not wish to talk at length about their problems, nor to find out about tests and treatment in any detail. Thirty-four of the 91 people interviewed thought stress and trying too hard could be a reason for fertility problems, and that talking about the problem would amplify this:

If you're relaxed, you're more likely to fall pregnant. It could be with Elaine, there's nothing wrong with her and the only reason she's not falling is because she's so fraught about it.

We don't go to bed saying tonight we're going to make a baby . . . I'm just trying to carry on as best I can and forget about it, and hopefully it will happen.

It's a vicious circle, if you start to worry about your periods. I think sometimes I wish I didn't have to watch myself so closely, taking my temperature.

The causes they gave were generally tentative, and counter-examples were often given, for example Tony's wife commented on his weight, but he retorted that men twice his size had families. Generally causation is not well established in subfertility, and it was rarely discussed at the clinics. In some medical conditions, as Fitzpatrick and Hopkins (1983, 308) have noted, personal knowledge is built up by painful trial and error; however, many subfertile people are symptom-free with no way of knowing, for example, whether bathing the testicles with cold water is improving the sperm count or not. Replies to questions about remedies showed a heavy reliance on medical expertise, and a tendency to caricature alternative medicine with reference to old wives' tales, although alternative approaches such as hypnotherapy have been used.

Unwillingness to find out more was unexpected, since studies of health care in Britain generally indicate that people want more information (Broome and Wallace 1984). American studies confirm this (e.g. Sandelowski, Harris and Holditch-Davis 1989), and the literature on health behaviour would have predicted that the people interviewed in this study would be well-informed 'consumers'. Many were middle-class, and would therefore be expected to have a greater knowledge of health matters (Townsend and Davidson 1982) and a notion of the body as 'something to be maintained and monitored' (Radley and Green 1987, 201). Women are also expected to take greater responsibility for health care and health knowledge (Graham 1984, Martin 1987). Several men and women had read a general health encyclopaedia, browsed through a book on fertility problems at bookstores, or read women's magazines, but it went no further than that:

> I read an article about childless couples – I can't remember a word of it! I don't get paranoid about it and read everything that I find. I wouldn't have bought a book though I might now we're on the treadmill.

> I haven't delved into it that deeply, I've left that to the specialist. If I dwelt on it, I'd become a hypochondriac.

> I don't think I would be very keen if you gave me a book now on 101 reasons for infertility. It would be like on your bad days you read a medical dictionary. I think that would just make me more neurotic about it.

For many couples, the strategy with most chance of success was to attend the clinic, take any prescribed drugs, and otherwise try to banish the problem from their day to day concerns. This strategy also underlay their feelings about self-help organisations. Only six of the 50 couples had either joined or thought that they might. Generally they did not see a self-help group as having any role other than discussion; 'just a group of people talking'; 'alright if you want that kind of thing, if you're desperate'; 'if the hospital can't help us, no-one can'. Since the couples in this study did not regard themselves as sub-fertile, but as parents-in-waiting, the self-help groups had the same stigma as the divorcees' club described by Hart (1976, 221); the aim was to help them adjust to a condition with which they did not wish to be associated, and from which they were trying to escape. In this they differed from Sandelowski's (1988) subfertile women, who did seek out other women with fertility problems.

Parents-in-Waiting

In my study, the majority had taken it for granted that they would become parents, and compared themselves to others in their social group (Salmon 1985):

> Chris' sister has just become pregnant – the worst thing on her mind was trying to tell me and Chris. Circumstances being what they are, the oldest one in the family usually has the baby first. All of Chris' life, Chris has always done everything first. I know it sounds a bit childish, but we got the first of everything.

> When I went to see my sister in hospital, I got upset, being younger than me. It was much easier with Pam [sister in law] because she was older than me. Being younger than me, for a few minutes I thought that should be me, not her.

Their answers indicated a broad consensus over what constitutes a 'normal' middle-class life-plan, in which couples use contraception for several years until secure housing and basic household equipment are obtained, and the couple feel they know each other (Jackson 1983, May 1982, Mansfield 1982, Owens 1986). They also felt that they should be 'mature' enough to cope with children, yet young enough to enjoy them:

> When you get to thirty, you're getting on a bit. If you're too old, you lose patience.

Twenty interviewees, both men and women, referred to their own or others' experiences as the child of older parents who were generally seen as less active, less able to empathise and rather an embarrassment to the schoolchild, who wants to be like everyone else. Motherhood is limited by the biological limits of menarche and menopause (although for the minority egg donation is changing the latter). Jackson (1983, 38) claims that 'men's vista of fertility is endless', but for the men in this study, the limits placed on fatherhood concerned the ability to be active; football in the park figured highly in their imagery of fatherhood. Lee, who had several young nieces and nephews when he was a teenager, was the most explicit of the men:

> There's just so much you can share with a kid. I suppose it's just going back to your own childhood again, you can be child with them. I love to cuddle little babies. When they're just born, they're so nice, and when they get a little bit older, you can be a little kid, and when they go to school you can help them, play football with them, then they grow up and you can go down the pub with them, they're friends. I'd give up anything to have a kid.

Children were not, however, viewed sentimentally or unrealistically, and people often resented well-meaning comments from their friends that they were well off without children:

They give you so much joy, so much love, something to share together between the two. They give you so much fun and enjoyment, even the 'orrible ones are great! I'd probably turn out with the liveliest little punk vandal you've ever seen!

I never get involved with other people's kids. I'm not interested – they're 'orrible things, to be quite honest. If they could be born at five, that would be great.

The longer you go without children, the more difficult it is to accept that they are going to ruin stuff.

Many were revising their expectations as time elapsed:

For all I know I could still be trying for a baby at 40, but I wouldn't let that stop me, because my life wouldn't be complete without children.

The determination to keep trying can curtail other options; although age limits on adoption have recently been lifted in the UK, at the time of this study they were quite strict, and for various reasons few couples favoured adoption. The lack of symptoms or clear-cut results to tests left many feeling in a state of limbo:

It wouldn't be so bad if there was something radically wrong with you like blocked tubes or something of that nature. Something physical. You could get to grips with it and perhaps circumvent it by test tube babies or whatever. But when there's nothing physically wrong with you, its just a little bit of hormone imbalance, and it's a hit and miss affair, that's what's so terribly frustrating.

We've gone full circle. We've learned a lot on the way, we've gained a lot in that respect. But I'm back with the very problem I first went with. One month with AID and there's an infection. That's been sorted out, the tubes have been opened, and we're back with the first problem. It just goes on and on.

That's it, that's the last test I shall do. I'm not going round in circles again. I'd rather go back on the pill and know I won't get pregnant; but to me, I think perhaps if I went back on the pill and came off it again, then perhaps I'd fall.

Most couples in this study coped by avoiding thinking about the future; as in Woollett's (1985) study, the focus changed from having a child to the finite time span of ovulation and menstruation.

The Marital Relationship

Much of the literature produced by the two voluntary groups refers to the considerable interpersonal tension generated by treatment; the word 'treadmill' is often used. The data on marital satisfaction is not clearcut, and psychological studies indicate rather confusing results (Callan 1987). Berger (1980), Connolly, Edelmann and Cooke (1987) and Feuer (1983) state that the sexual relationship is particularly disrupted when the man has a fertility problem, although data from Humphrey (1983) indicate that impotence is not a great problem. Humphrey (1969) and Owens (1982) also think that the man is more stigmatised. Many couples who had been in treatment for over a year reported that they had become closer, but at considerable cost:

He got in from the pub and I told him my temperature had gone up.
    I don't care who you are, I cannot just, my temperature's gone up, go up there and perform, and I will not do that just because a chart, we've done all that before, and we've had more rows than anything. I'd rather say right, I'll not have a kid, than do things like that. Because to me that should be natural, not bloody set out.

We never fell out – just a strain on our sex life. It didn't draw us closer together that we cling to each other, and it certainly didn't push us further apart. We try to keep things as normal as possible.

You have to laugh, you'd go mad, wouldn't you? It's like the douche, it says five minutes before. It takes you five minutes to get upstairs from the bathroom!

It might sound funny like, a lot of people say to have a good marriage you've got to have problems to bring you together. That's marriage, isn't it, 'cos you're partners.

Talking to Others

Some of the stress which couples experienced could perhaps have been reduced by obtaining emotional support from other family members or friends. Forty of the 50 couples had told their parents they were attending a clinic, mainly because they felt they should know why they were not being made grandparents. Several realised they might have to visit the clinic frequently, and rather than 'play MI5' and invent excuses for visits to London, it was better to 'come clean'. Generally, however, clinic attendance was not a topic of conversation. Marriage and parenthood problems in the UK are generally regarded as best coped with by the couple themselves (Pearlin and Schooler 1978, Woollett 1985), and parents were reluctant to 'pry'. It should also be noted that, despite the counselling literature which emphasises the value of talking (see below), the evidence is equivocal. Emotional distancing may sometimes be the best policy (Folkman and Lazarus 1988), and talking may increase, rather than reduce, depression (Ross and Mirowsky 1989). For a minority of couples their parents had no other grandchildren, and had their own grief and disappointment (Shapiro 1982):

> My father, I think he's taken it badly, and he doesn't talk about it to my mum. I seem to able to talk to him better over the phone about it than actually speaking face to face, because I do find I get a bit emotional about it . . . I do feel guilty. I did say well there's a bit of hope, but I don't want to say too much because I don't want their hopes to rise.

AID is a particularly sensitive issue. Four couples in this study were involved in AID and one was contemplating it; two had told one set of parents, and three had told neither, confirming findings in larger studies by Humphrey (1983) and Snowden and Snowden (1984).

Being Different

A minority of interviewees (12 women, six men) indicated in their discussion that they felt in some way 'odd' or incomplete:

> Yes, you've failed again. Not just in the purely medical sense, as a person. I feel guilty. There's no reason why you should feel guilty, because you haven't done anything wrong. Maybe it's a feeling of failure as a human being. I've thought about it recently. I was looking at a Reject Shop, where you buy very good quality goods with very good beginnings, but something went wrong along the way. They've become rejects. I found myself comparing myself along those terms. It sounds a bit nutty perhaps.

Attendance at the clinic did not seem to mark any kind of transition point to a patient identity, as claimed by Stanway (1980) and some of the American studies (Sandelowski and Pollock 1986, Olshansky 1987). However, two-thirds of the women and eight of the men interviewed experienced some feelings of discomfort, particularly around the situation of others' pregnancies:

> I got angry because everyone was worried about me, sort of taking it away from Jenny [sister in law]. It's only because people care, but sometimes it's nice to be treated like a normal person. So I went shopping and bought her a panda thing. She only works across the road in the bank. It took me all my strength of will – I know it sounds silly – and I thought I hope you're not there Jenny, and she wasn't. So I left it with someone. It was my way of saying I'm pleased for you.

> The unforgivable thing was Pete and Ann, when she first fell pregnant. D'you know, she was pregnant for three months before she told us, and everyone in my family knew she was pregnant, and they wouldn't. In the end my mum came round and told us. I was really upset, because Pete was

like a brother. I told him how hurt I was. D'you think that would upset us? We're pleased for you. It's more upsetting to be told weeks after everyone else. That really made us feel lonely social outcasts.

Generally, the announcement of a wanted pregnancy should be greeted with pleasure by all hearers, especially women. If it is known that the person who is about to hear the news has been trying unsuccessfully for a child, however, it can seem tactless to be too cheerful. The announcer can carry on as usual, although this may be hurtful, or avoid the situation, which is even more hurtful because special consideration can be subtly degrading (Baruch 1982, 204–205, Locker 1982). Many childless women also feel uneasy when asked by casual acquaintances if they have children. It is often asked in a spirit of polite enquiry, expecting the answer 'yes', and 'no' leaves a hole in the conversational fabric which requires repair work. The originator of the question is not, however, expecting to hear of some personal problem, and may feel they have committed a *faux pas*:

I say I've had an ectopic, but then people think 'Oh my God, what did I ask'?

Few described situations of ribald teasing such as occurred in Miall's (1985) Canadian study, and they were met with good humour. A more pervasive feeling, especially from women who had attended the clinic for several years, was that of drifting away from friends as the latter found their time and attention consumed by parenthood:

I work hard at not being left out. I don't exclude myself from conversations about children. I talk in a way that I appear very interested – I hope. But I'm more and more aware of being excluded from that world.

The overall picture obtained in my study was that couples experienced some strain on their relationship and felt different from others. Those who had been in treatment for some time were conscious of time running out, although they tried not to become too 'obsessed' with the problem, and this deterred them from finding out more about it. They did not believe that talking about it would help very much, and discussion was limited in the clinics.

Implications for Nursing Care

As the previous discussion has indicated, the research on the experience of subfertility does not give a clear-cut picture; there may be cultural differences between the US and the UK, as well as differences in the health care systems, which account for some of this. In general, the American data are more dramatic and portray the woman as an active health care consumer who embarks on treatment as a career; the man is less involved, since parenthood is not his central role in life. A further body of literature, produced by social workers and counsellors, draws on bereavement models (Shapiro 1982, Daniels 1992, Menning 1980, Valentine 1986), whereas the people in both my own and Owens' (1986) study did not generally suffer from a bereavement as such, since they continued to see themselves as parents-in-waiting. The concept of chronic sorrow, which is interwoven with periods of neutrality and happiness, may be more useful in subfertility than that of bereavement (Teal 1991). It is important not to make assumptions about how people feel; it is also important that, whenever possible, the couple is given the opportunity to explore their feelings together, and it is recognised that these feelings may not coincide.

Issues for nursing assessment include the following:

- How long have the couple been in treatment, and at what stage do they perceive themselves to be?
- Do they need further information?
- What coping mechanisms do they use? These may include emotion management, information gathering, or comparison with others who are less fortunate.
- What health beliefs do they have about the causes and treatment of subfertility?
- Are there any situations which are particularly difficult?

One aspect of assessment which is not appropriate for nurses is that of assessing whether the couple are suited for parenting, as advocated by the HFEA; it is probably best carried out by someone not directly involved in the treatment process.

Nursing Problems

Based on the information gathered, these may include the following:

- Stress caused either by the treatment process, or the social effects of subfertility, such as feelings of isolation. Stress is likely to be particularly acute for women undergoing IVF or GIFT, since they have a particular event on which to pin their hopes (Greenfeld, Diamond and Decherney 1988, Leiblum et al 1987)
- Women (or more rarely men) undergoing surgery may have anxieties about the effects of anaesthesia, or postoperative pain.
- Anxiety and uncertainty about outcomes, and the awareness of time passing.
- Disturbance in self-concept, particularly for the woman.
- Possible marital disharmony.
- Feelings of guilt, or not wanting to burden the other partner.
- If the individual shows preoccupation, depression or uncontrollable emotion, counselling should be suggested (Daniels 1992).

Planning and Implementation

The major goal should be that the couple emerge from treatment having succeeded in having a child, or in coming to terms with their subfertility and able to make alternative plans. If they do not conceive it is important that they feel able to stop treatment, rather than persist *ad infinitum*; Sandelowski et al (1989) describe the subfertile as 'intolerant of regret', fearful that they may look back and think 'if only we had persisted, we might have succeeded'.

Counselling

Counselling is a specific issue in subfertility, since it must be offered by law in the UK in licensed clinics under the HFEA. There are three types of counselling specified: implications of treatment, support and therapeutic. There is a debate about whether nurses are able to take the role of counsellor, since some writers maintain that they may be too involved with the physical aspects of treatment (Hunt 1992, Inglis and Denton 1992, Daniels 1992) and that social workers or psychologists should undertake counselling. A survey of the Fertility Nursing Group of the Royal College of Nursing (1990) found that in more than half the units surveyed nurses were the main counsellors, but only half of these had had training; this issue is taken up by the King's Fund report, Counselling for Regulated Fertility Treatments (1991). A diploma in fertility counselling was set up at the Royal London Hospital in 1989, led by Dr Sue Jennings, and the Institute of Advanced Nursing Education is currently developing a course in fertility nursing. However, we need to know more about what couples want, as opposed to what we think they need. Inglis (1992) has found in her IVF work that 60 per cent of couples take up counselling, but only 12 per cent wish to have counselling in depth, and prior to IVF they require support, not counselling.

Other Roles

Fertility nursing is an area where there is a wide variety of roles; Lady Diana Brittan, deputy chair of the HFEA, regards the nurse's coordinator role in clinics as pivotal. The UKCC Scope for Professional Practice document, which signals a move from certification for specific tasks to broad general principles, enables nurses to undertake embryo transfers (e.g. in Oxford), and transvaginal scanning for follicular development to time AID. Practitioners feel that this enhances continuity of care, and professional indemnification through the RCN is now possible, provided that the unit has an assessed training scheme and a protocol.

Conclusion

The main conclusion to this chapter is that fertility treatment covers a wide spectrum in which nurses may play a central role. Many treatments are not successful, however, and the social aspects of fertility problems are as important as the medical and nursing treatments. It is therefore important that we as nurses try to keep abreast with the debates surrounding these controversial treatments, and that we do not underestimate the pain of being different.

Acknowledgements

I would like to acknowledge the help of the following in writing this chapter: Jane Denton, Chairman of the RCN Fertility Nurses Group, Angela Lumsdon of Serono, Margaret Inglis and Anna Brophy.

References

Abdalla H, Baber R and Studd J (1990) Active management of infertility. In Studd J (ed.) *Progress in Obstetrics and Gynaecology*, Vol 8. Edinburgh: Churchill Livingstone.

Allan G A (1980) A note on interviewing spouses together. *Journal of Marriage and the Family*, **42**, February, 205–10.

Allison J R (1979) Role and role conflict of women in infertile couples. *Psychology of Women Quarterly*, **4**, 1, 97–113.

Baluch B, Manyande A and Aghssa M A (1993) *Failure to conceive with in vitro fertilisation: the Middle Eastern experience*. Unpublished paper.

Baruch G (1982) *Moral tales: interviewing parents of congenitally ill children*. Unpublished PhD Thesis, University of London.

Baum F (1980) *Childless by choice: a sociological study of a demographic phenomenon in Britain*. Unpublished PhD Thesis, University of Nottingham.

Berger D (1980) Impotence following the discovery of azoospermia. *Fertility and Sterility*, **34**, 154–156.

Broome A and Wallace L (1984) *Psychology and Gynaecological Problems*. London: Tavistock.

Busfield J and Paddon M (1977) *Thinking about Children*. London: Cambridge University Press.

Callan V (1987) The personal and marital adjustment of mothers and of voluntarily and involuntarily childless wives. *Journal of Marriage and the Family*, **49**, February, 847–856.

Campbell E (1985) *The Childless Marriage*. London: Tavistock.

Connolly K, Edelmann R and Cooke I (1987) Distress and marital problems associated with infertility. *Journal of Reproductive and Infant Psychology*, **5**, 49–57.

Cooper S (1979) *Female infertility: its effect on self esteem, body image, locus of control, and behavior*. Unpublished PhD Thesis, Boston University.

Corea G (1985) *The Mother Machine*. London: The Women's Press.

Daniels K (1992) Management of the psychological aspects of infertility. *Australian & New Zealand Journal of Obstetrics and Gynaecology*, **32**, 1, 57–63.

Dixon J and Gilbert Welch J (1991) Priority setting: lessons from Oregon. *Lancet*, **337**, 891–894.

Elias N (1985) *The Loneliness of the Dying*. Oxford: Basil Blackwell.

Emerson J (1970a) Nothing unusual is happening. In Shibutani T (ed.) *Human Nature and Collective Behavior*. Englewood Cliffs: Prentice Hall.

Emerson J (1970b) Behavior in private places: sustaining definitions of reality in gynecological examinations. In Dreitzel H (ed.) *Recent Sociology*. New York: Macmillan.

Entwistle P (1992) Is pregnancy the only success story in infertility. *Conceive*, **23**, August, 10.

Fertility Nursing Group (1990) Report of a professional survey. London: RCN.

Feuer G (1983) *The psychological impact of infertility on the lives of men*. Unpublished PhD Thesis, University of Pennsylvania.

Fitzpatrick R and Hopkins A (1983) Problems in the conceptual framework of patient satisfaction research: an empirical exploration. *Sociology of Health and Illness*, **5**, 3, 297–311.

Folkman S and Lazarus R (1988) The relationship between coping and emotion: implications for theory and research. *Social Science and Medicine*, **26**, 3, 309–317.

Franklin S (1990) Deconstructing 'desperateness': the social construction of infertility in popular representations of new reproductive technologies. In McNeil M, Varcoe I and Yearley S (eds) *The New Reproductive Technologies*. London: Macmillan.

Goffman E (1974) *Frame Analysis*. Harmondsworth: Penguin.

Graham H (1984) *Women, Health and the Family*. Brighton: Wheatsheaf.

Greenfeld D, Diamond M and Decherney A (1988) Grief reactions following in vitro fertilisation treatment. *Journal of Psychosomatic Obstetrics and Gynaecology*, **8**, 169–174.

Greil A, Leitko T and Porter K (1988) Infertility: his and hers. *Gender and Society*, **2**, 2, 172–199.

Harding S (1988) Trends in permissiveness. In Jowell R et al (eds) *British Social Attitudes: the 5th Report*. Aldershot: Gower.

Harman H (1990) *Trying for a Baby: a Report on the Inadequacy of NHS Infertility Services*. House of Commons.

Hart N (1976) *When Marriage Ends*. London: Tavistock.

Henslin J and Biggs M (1971) Dramaturgical desexualisation: the sociology of the vaginal examination. In Henslin J (ed.) *Studies in the Sociology of Sex*. New York: Appleton Century Crofts.

Heywood A (1991) Immaculate conception? *Nursing Times*, **87**, 22, 62–63.

Hirsch M and Mosher W (1987) Characteristics of infertile women in the United States and their use of fertility services. *Fertility and Sterility*, **47**, 4, 618–625.

Houghton P and Houghton D (1977) *Unfocussed Grief*. Birmingham Settlement.

Houghton P and Houghton D (1984) *Coping with Childlessness*. London: George Allan & Unwin.

Hull M (1985) Infertility – its extent and nature. *Conceive*, **1**, April.

Human Fertilisation and Embryology Authority (1992) Annual Report. London.

Humphrey M (1969) *The Hostage Seekers*. London: Longman.

Humphrey M (1975) The effect of children upon the marriage relationship. *British Journal of Medical Psychology*, **48**, 273–279.

Humphrey M (1983) Paper given at NAC meeting, Isleworth.

Hunt J (1992) *The role of counselling in licenced and nonlicenced centres*. Paper given at Serono Seminar, Counselling Skills and Fertility Management, York, September.

Hunt M and Meerabeau E (1993) Purging the emotions: the lack of emotional expression in subfertility and in the care of the dying. *International Journal of Nursing Studies*, **30**, 2, 115–123.

Inglis M (1992) Personal communication.

Inglis M and Denton J (1992) Infertility nurses and counselling. In Templeton A and Drife J (eds) *Infertility*. London: Springer-Verlag.

Jackson B (1983) *Fatherhood*. London: George Allan & Unwin.

King's Fund Centre Counselling Committee (1991) Counselling for regulated fertility treatments. London: King's Fund.

Lawler J (1991) *Behind the Screens: Nursing, Somology and the Problem of the Body*. Melbourne: Churchill Livingstone.

Leiblum S, Kemman E, Colburn D, Pasquale S and De Lisi A (1987) Unsuccessful in vitro fertilisation: a follow up study. *Journal of In Vitro Fertilisation and Embryo Transfer*, **4**, 1, 46–50.

Lewis C and O'Brien M (1987) *Reassessing Fatherhood: New Observations on Fathers and the Modern Family*. London: Sage.

Locker D (1983) *Disability and Disadvantage: the Consequences of Chronic Illness*. London: Tavistock.

Mansfield P (1982) Getting ready for parenthood: attitudes to and expectations of having children of a group of newly weds. *International Journal of Social Policy*, **2**, 28–29.

Martin E (1987) *The Woman in the Body: a Cultural Analysis of Reproduction*. New York: Beacon Press.

Mathieson D (1986) *Infertility Services in the NHS: What's Going On?* Report prepared for Frank Dobson, MP.

May K (1982) Factors contributing to first time fathers' readiness for fatherhood. *Family Relations*, **31**, 353–362.

McGilvray D (1982) Sexual power and fertility in Sri Lanka. In McCormack C (ed.) *Ethnography of Fertility and Birth*. London: Academic Press.

McNeil M, Varcoe I and Yearly S (1990) The New Reproductive Technologies. London: Macmillan.

Meerabeau E (1991) Husbands' participation in fertility treatment: they also serve who only stand and wait. *Sociology of Health and Illness*, **13**, 3, 396–410.

Menning B (1980) The emotional needs of infertile people. *Fertility and Sterility*, **43**, 313–319.

Miall C (1985) Perceptions of informal sanctioning and the stigma of involuntary childlessness. *Deviant Behavior*, **6**, 383–403.

Montague A (1991) Avoiding misconceptions. *Guardian*, 19.7.91.

Ng C, Tsakok F, Tan S and Chan K (eds) (1988) *Frontiers in Reproductive Endocrinology and Infertility*. Dordrecht: Kluwer Academic Publishers.

Olshansky E (1987) Identity of self as infertile: an example of theory generating research. *Advances in Nursing Science*, **9**, 2, 54–63.

Owens D (1982) The desire to father: reproductive ideologies and involuntarily childless men. In McKee L and O'Brien M (eds) *The Father Figure*. London: Tavistock.

Owens D (1986) *The desire for children: a sociological study of involuntary childlessness*. Unpublished PhD Thesis, University College, Cardiff.

Pearlin L and Schooler C (1978) The structure of coping. *Journal of Health and Social Behaviour*, **19**, 2–21.

Pfeffer N (1987a) Artificial insemination, in vitro fertilisation and the stigma of infertility. In Stanworth M (ed.) *Reproductive Technologies: Gender, Motherhood and Medicine*. Oxford: Basil Blackwell/Polity Press.

Pfeffer N (1987b) *Pronatalism and sterility 1900–50*. Unpublished PhD Thesis, University of Essex.

Pfeffer N and Quick A (1988) *Infertility Services: a Desperate Case*. London, GLACHC.

Pfeffer N and Woollett A (1983) *The Experience of Infertility*. London: Virago.

Radley A and Green R (1987) Illness as adjustment: a methodology and conceptual framework. *Sociology of Health and Illness*, **9**, 2, 179–207.

Ross C and Mirowsky J (1989) Explaining the social patterns of depression: control and problem solving – or support and talking? *Journal of Health and Social Behaviour*, 30, June, 206–219.

Salmon P (1985) *Living in Time*. London: JM Dent & Sons.

Sandelowski M (1988) Without child: the world of infertile women. *Health Care for Women International*, **9**, 147–161.

Sandelowski M and Pollock C (1986) Women's experience of infertility. *Image: Journal of Nursing Scholarship*, **18**, 4, 140–144.

Sandelowski M, Harris B and Holditch-Davis D (1989) Mazing: infertile couples and the quest for a child. *Image: Journal of Nursing Scholarship*, **21**, 4, 220–226.

Scully P and Bart P (1973) A funny thing happened on the way to the orifice: women in gynecology textbooks. *American Journal of Sociology*, **78**, 4, 1045–1049.

Seibel M (1990) *Infertility: a Comprehensive Text*. Norwalk: Appleton & Lange.

Shapiro C (1982) The impact of infertility on the marital relationship. *Social Casework*, **63**, 7, 387–393.

Snowden R and Snowden E (1984) *The Gift of a Child*. London: George Allan & Unwin.

Snowden R, Mitchell G and Snowden E (1983) *Artificial Reproduction: a Sociological Investigation*. London: George Allan & Unwin.

Stacey M (ed.) (1992) *Changing Human Reproduction*. London: Sage.

Stanway A (1980) *Why Us?* London: Granada.

Strickler J (1992) Reproductive technology: problem or solution? *Sociology of Health and Illness*, **14**, 1, 111–132.

Strong P (1979) *The Ceremonial Order of the Clinic: Parents, Doctors and Medical Bureaucracies*. London: Routledge & Kegan Paul.

Teal C (1991) Chronic sorrow: an analysis of the concept. *Journal of Advanced Nursing*, **16**, 11, 1311–1319.

Thomas T and Heberton B (1991) Tin opener for a can of worms. *Health Service Journal*, 8 August, 21.

Townsend P and Davidson N (1982) *Inequalities in Health*. Harmondsworth: Penguin.

Valentine D (1986) Psychological impact of infertility: identifying issues and needs. *Social Work in Health Care*, **11**, 4, 61–69.

Veevers J (1979) Voluntary childlessness: a review of issues and evidence. *Marriage and Family Review*, **2**, 2, 1–26.

Warnock M (1984) *A Question of Life*. Oxford: Basil Blackwell.

Winston R (1986) *Infertility: a Sympathetic Approach*. London: Martin Dunitz.

Woollett A (1985) Childlessness: strategies for coping with infertility. *International Journal of Behavioural Development*, **8**, 473–482.

Woollett A (1991) Having children: accounts of childless women and women with reproductive problems. In Phoenix A, Woollett A and Lloyd E (eds) *Motherhood: Meanings, Practices and Ideologies*. London: Sage.

Chapter 3
Young Men's Experiences of Testicular Cancer
Liz Jones and Christine Webb

Introduction

Testicular cancer is currently probably the most successfully treatable of all the solid malignant tumours. Medical management of this disease represents one of the biggest success stories in the history of cancer treatment. But what are the experiences of men who are affected by this condition? Medical and nursing optimism may obscure what the disease experience means to them. Could it be that, as a young man with Hodgkin's disease comments:

> To the oncologist, an 80 per cent cure rate for Hodgkin's disease may look impressive. To the patient it may look more like a one in five chance of impending death.
>
> (Cooper 1982, 613)

In this chapter we will discuss issues related to sexuality emerging from a study of young men with testicular cancer carried out by Liz Jones, and consider their implications for nursing care. The scene will be set by reviewing previous research on the topic.

The Medical and Psychosocial Background

The vast majority of testicular cancers arise from the germ cells of the testis. The overall incidence of the disease in the UK is 3.8 per 100,000, which accounts for only 2 per cent of all male cancers. However, the incidence in men between 25 and 34 years rises to 9.4 per 100,000 and testicular cancer is the most common form of cancer in young men between 20 and 34 years, with approximately 900 new cases occurring each year in the UK (Office of Population Censuses and Surveys 1985). It is also important that the incidence is increasing and has almost doubled over the last 20 years (Peckham 1988, Horwich 1991).

The aetiology of testicular cancer remains unclear except that there is an increased incidence in men with a history of testicular maldescent. However, even then only 10 per cent of men with testicular cancer have a history of cryptorchidism (Pike, Chilvers and Peckham 1986, Senturia 1987).

The prognosis of testicular cancer has greatly improved over the last 20 years. Before 1970 most men with metastatic disease died (Blandy, Hope-Stone and Dayan 1970, Peckham 1988), but today the cure rate is well over 90 per cent. Even in the few cases where men present with widespread disease, the cure rate is still very high.

The reasons that medical management has improved so dramatically are the development of highly accurate methods of diagnosis, monitoring of progress and effective chemotherapy. However, treatments can lead to unwanted effects. Following orchidectomy, Hendry et al (1983) have found that many men either have very low sperm counts or that no viable sperm are identifiable, although fertility may recover spontaneously. Chemotherapy and radiotherapy treatments will render the man sterile at the time, but for a proportion this also has been found to be a temporary effect (Horwich 1991).

Testicular cancer affects men at a time in their lives when they are building careers, relationships and families, and when sexual activity is generally considered to be an important aspect of their lives as young men. It therefore seems reasonable to assume that cancer of the testis will have quite an impact on sexuality in all its facets.

There has been little nursing research into this subject, the only British study being an investigation of the impact of orchidectomy upon sexuality (Blackmore 1988). A few nursing studies have been carried out in the USA, but care is needed in relating their findings to the UK situation because of cultural and medical management differences.

Several studies carried out recently, mostly in the USA but also in Europe, have investigated the psychosocial aspects of testicular cancer and long-term survival (see, for example, Loescher et al 1990, Kaasa et al 1991, Hannah et al 1992, Douchez et al 1993).

Topics investigated include psychosexual issues, fertility, effects on intimate relationships and psychological and social effects. Some contradictory findings have emerged, but it seems reasonable to conclude that for some people the experience of having testicular cancer has positive effects, for example on marital relationships or outlook on life. Conclusions from studies looking at sexual and fertility issues vary, but it seems that for a minority of men these can be a source of distress. Long-term psychosocial effects also vary, with some studies reporting mood disturbances, particularly higher levels of anxiety and fear concerning disease recurrence.

A retrospective study of psychosocial problems experienced by testicular cancer patients and their relatives has been undertaken by Moynihan, a British psychologist (Moynihan 1987). She reports that men's worries are not static, but change over the course of the disease and its treatment, and this has important implications for care at different stages in the cancer experience.

Orchidectomy is performed both for diagnosis and as the primary (and in some cases only) treatment for testicular cancer, but there is little evidence of its psychosocial effects. In a small study, Blackmore (1988) found no significant differences in sexual functioning when comparing 16 men who had had orchidectomy for testicular cancer with 5 who had had orchidectomy for non-malignant causes and 10 with no history of testicular problems. However, it emerged from the study that some men in all three groups had sexual problems and that a proportion of men with testicular cancer did perceive a difference in their own sexual drive after surgery. Blackmore concludes that sexual problems occur throughout the population and that some men with testicular cancer may have had pre-existing sexual problems and may attribute these to their diagnosis or treatment.

However, Rieker, Edbril and Garnick (1985), exploring sexual functioning in men who had been cured of testicular cancer, found the greatest impairment and substantially more psychological distress in men who tended to conceal their emotions. The authors suggest that this may be a group of men who hold traditional ideas about male behaviour and in particular do not disclose emotions. It may also be that for this group sexual performance is more closely linked with definitions of 'manliness'.

In the American and European studies (Rieker et al 1985), psychological distress related to sexual functioning appears to be very much more important than in British reports (Moynihan 1987, Stuart et al 1990). This may be explainable by differences in medical management. Retroperitoneal lymphadenectomy, which frequently causes ejaculatory dysfunction, is standard medical management for early stage disease in the USA and Europe. However, in the UK this is usually only used when there are signs of residual disease after other treatments have been given. Another possible explanation of differences in psychological distress related to sexual functioning lies in cultural differences between countries.

Several studies report that the experience of testicular cancer affects intimate relationships. Rieker et al (1985) found that 68 per cent of marriages were reported to be strengthened and 32 per cent strained, whereas 26 per cent of lover relationships were strengthened and 74 per cent were strained.

Employment appears to be a more important issue for men with testicular cancer in the UK than in the USA. Moynihan (1987) and Stuart et al (1990) both report a greater risk of unemployment and loss of job prospects, which are an important cause of psychological distress.

Finally, outlook on life seems to be an important influence. Studies of men who have survived testicular cancer report a higher number of perceived health worries than would be expected in the general population, with a high frequency of any physical symptom being attributed to recurrence of the cancer. Studies by Kennedy et al (1976), Rieker et al (1985), Cassileth and Steinfeld (1987) and Stuart et al (1990) suggest strongly that the experience of cancer in general is reported as having some very positive aspects. Many survivors perceive that their lives have been improved, that they have had an opportunity to reassess their priorities in life, and that surviving the disease in itself is an accomplishment.

In summary, men's experiences of testicular cancer are a neglected area of study by nurses. As a result, information on which to base care is lacking and it is possible that distress could be diminished if staff were able to be more aware of potentially important issues and be more supportive. Therefore it was decided to study young men's experiences of testicular cancer.

The Study

The aims of the study were as follows.

1. To explore the experiences and feelings of men with testicular cancer and their interpretations as these developed over time.
2. To assist nurses in their understanding of men's experiences, thus facilitating the delivery of appropriate care.

The original impetus for the study came from Liz Jones' experiences as a nurse caring for men with this disease and her realisation that on one hand they were part of a big medical success story, but on the other hand she had little idea of what the illness experience entailed for them. Therefore it was appropriate to use an exploratory approach to the research, and to conduct unstructured interviews in which men were asked to talk openly and freely about whatever aspects they themselves wanted and thought important. The role of Liz Jones as interviewer was to encourage and facilitate their story-telling, but not to impose any outside agenda.

Eighteen men between the ages of 20 and 40 years were recruited from a specialist cancer hospital and all interviews took place in the men's homes, except one which was conducted at the interviewer's place of work for the convenience of the participant.

Thirteen men were interviewed once only, three were interviewed on two occasions, and three were interviewed three times. All first interviews occurred within four months of diagnosis and any further interviews were within the first year. Seven men were interviewed with their partners present for some or all of the time. All interviews were tape-recorded and transcribed verbatim, and preliminary analysis for major themes was undertaken throughout the process of data collection. Further analysis was completed after all interviews were finished.

The idea of a journey or career has developed as the overall theme linking participants' different accounts of their experiences. The main stages in this journey, reported in the men's own words, are:

1. *Getting it sorted* – the start of the problem.
2. *It was a bombshell at first* – response to diagnosis.
3. *It didn't really worry me as long as it took everything with it when it went* – thoughts about removal of testis.
4. *You're all right, the left one's still there* – thoughts about sexual functioning.
5. *Kids are about the last thing on my mind at the moment* – thoughts about fertility.

6. *In limbo* – waiting for results and further treatment.
7. *On chemo* – treatment experiences.
8. *Light at the end of the tunnel* – after treatment and follow-up.

In this chapter we will discuss aspects linked to sexuality by focusing on stages 3, 4 and 5 concerning testicular loss, sexual functioning and fertility.

It Didn't Really Worry Me as Long as it Took Everything With it When it Went

Men's thoughts about losing the testis seemed to be influenced by several aspects of their experiences.

Lack of information
This emerged as important in the study, with some men not realising that removal of the testis was not the end of the story, but was just the first stage in their management and that they would need follow-up and perhaps further treatment in a specialist cancer hospital.

One of their primary sources of information was the surgeon who performed the operation in their local district general hospital. For three men, information about the curability of the cancer was given to them at the same time as they were told about the need for orchidectomy. As a result they believed that surgery was the complete treatment, and their later referral to a specialist hospital caused shock and distress.

Much of the information they had received seemed brief and purely functional, such as 'it will have to come off' or that it is possible to function 'as well with one as with two'. According to the men's reports, it also seemed that some information received from surgeons was inaccurate regarding fertility and treatment options. Five men also said that they had been surprised by the site of the surgical incision, expecting the testis to be removed from the scrotum rather than via the abdomen.

Previous experiences had given some men knowledge of what to expect because three had undergone orchidopexy in childhood for cryptorchidism and two had had vasectomies. Other sources of information and reassurance were others who had had similar surgery and, in one case, a friend who was a medical student.

However, the fact that they had cancer, rather than removal of the testis, was the major concern for many men. Secondly, some men's fears focused on this being their first hospitalisation, surgery or anaesthetic. But the main issue was that they had a potentially life-threatening condition, as expressed by P11:

> It didn't really worry me, to be honest, losing it – no – as long as it took everything with it when it went.

Initial shock was the reaction of five men to the loss of their testis, but this was short-lived (P5):

> I suppose when I woke up groggily – the doctor came in – I'm lying flat on my back – and he told me, they told us what they'd done. I suppose it came as a shock. But then again you get a sense of relief that that's it – gone.

Many of the men went on to explain or rationalise why the loss of a testis is of little concern (P8):

> It was – it's of no consequence to me really . . . I mean it doesn't make any difference to the workings of anything. And aesthetically – I mean I – if anybody looks at me I've still got – I appear to have the normal equipment. Because I've still got the scrotum there, I've still got the sac there, and I do – I do notice it's missing, there's no doubt about it, but it's – it doesn't cause me any psychological problem whatsoever.

Some men described how glad they were to be rid of the testis as the source of the cancer (P1):

> I wasn't really that bothered about that actually. I wanted it to be gone. You know, I – I just wanted him to take it away. So I said to him, 'I don't care about anything else, just – just get me in the hospital and get it away.

Two men explained that the enlarged testis had been a cause of nuisance and discomfort, and they saw its removal in a positive light. Several, in describing how they thought about the orchidectomy, compared themselves to others and remarked that things could have been worse.

Whether or not they felt that they had undergone an *alteration in appearance* seemed to influence the men's reactions to testicular loss. The most frequently given reason for loss of the testis not being a problem was that this was not noticeable to others. Several men spontaneously compared their situation to that of a woman having a mastectomy (P15):

> I suppose it's similar to breast cancer in women, you know, only not quite as traumatic possibly . . . I'm only trying to – looking at it from a man's point of view. That, with a women, sort of the, you know, the breast side of it is more, if you like – fashion or whatever . . . Whereas with a man, you know, you couldn't tell, you know, that you have had one removed. And also you don't need, sort of, you know, false bras or – you know what I mean – it would be inhibiting for a woman . . . it would be very obvious and you'd probably be restricted . . . Whereas the operation I've had won't restrict me in doing anything 'normal' (in inverted commas); people would never know.

Some men were aware of a visible change but saw this as a positive thing because previously the testis had been abnormally enlarged and had caused discomfort. For example P8 and his wife discussed this point:

(P8)   I don't know whether you've – I mean you've obviously noticed that one's gone. But does it bother you at all?
(W8)   No, it doesn't. It doesn't bother me, no. And like you say, to look at it looks more normal now than it did for a long time before, sort of thing, really.
(P8)   . . . If I stand in the mirror and look at myself I look more normal now than I did before the operation . . . I could stand in the shower with a gang – with another gang of blokes, you know, who are all having a shower together, and I don't feel inadequate in any way, shape or form.

Some men stated that they were aware of the loss and change in appearance but that this was not a cause of concern. However, the two youngest men did show some concern about loss of the testis. P9 was particularly concerned in the first interview but by the second interview he stated that he was still aware of the absence but it no longer bothered him as there was nothing he could do about it. Indeed, on this occasion he seemed to be far more relaxed about the situation. In contrast P14, who was 20 years old, expressed little concern in the first interview but showed more ambivalence in the second (P14):

I don't think about it that often. Erm – it can be a bit embarrassing if you're swimming and things like that, when you're getting changed in front of other people . . . but nobody else knows and nobody cares but because you know, you think everybody else can tell. But they can't, but you think they can – [laughs] – and half of me thinks, well, yes, it's worrying, and the other half thinks, well – I don't care what they think – [laughs].

Interactions with other people

These were problematic for some men after their orchidectomy, because they were embarrassed about the site of the condition. P5 experienced embarrassment when a female neighbour enquired about why he had been in hospital, and P15 similarly found himself in a potentially embarrassing situation when asked about the nature of his surgery by fellow patients on a mixed-sex ward. P16 found that he did not want people he worked with to know about his illness because (P16):

Some people may know, but obviously . . . that I had it down there, really. I don't want people to look down there when they're talking to me . . .

Joking seemed to be one way of coping with interactions with others. Some men talked about the use of jokes between themselves and their partners or friends, or with doctors, or joked in the interviews. It seemed that joking was used to smooth over potentially difficult social situations.

Manhood

'Manhood' was a term used by some of the men when talking about whether or not they saw loss of a testis as altering their self-identity as a man. Two men said openly that they had feared that losing the testis would threaten their 'manhood' (P9):

It's, er, didn't make me feel any less a man at first. But I think just these last few weeks it's getting to me. Because I'm starting to feel that way, you know, that – it's just wrong. Just looks wrong and everything.

In the first interview P9 expressed the most distress by far on this point, but by the time of the second interview 6 months later his response was (P9):

It was starting to niggle me, you know, but now I think I just accept it. You know, it's as it's going to be, so that's it. Not a lot you can do about it.

When asked why he had first sought medical advice, P7 said:

I suppose basically underlying it all, I suppose, it's a fear of a man losing his manhood, really.

Seven men stated very clearly and quite forcibly that they did not feel 'any less of a man' as a result of their testicular loss. P15 expressed it thus:

Daft as it may be – you know, um – I just knew that by taking it out it would help – well, I understood at that time it would solve that problem, so, you know, go ahead and do it. You know, he could have done it the next day as far as I was concerned . . . I didn't feel it was any threat, you know, to my manhood or anything.

P1 said:

Like those blokes who start thinking they're not – a full man. You know, maybe if I didn't think that I was still a whole – I still feel that I'm a full person. I don't feel that it makes any difference . . . I'm still me.

Possible spread to the other testis was something that did cause concern to seven men. P16 was particularly concerned when his second testis became enlarged, and bypassed his general practitioner to go straight to the surgeon the following day:

I thought the other one would have to come out. I was concerned obviously for losing the second testicle, but also at that time I was feeling very weak and a bit depressed, and to have to go through all that operation again, er, I wasn't – I don't know, you know, I just didn't think I could go through it.

It turned out that the problem with the other testis was an infection.

Loss of the testis in itself, then, had not been the predominant issue for most men. Their diagnosis of cancer had been what had worried them the most, and in many cases lack of information or even inaccurate information had added to their distress. Once the surgery was over, they were not usually troubled by a changed physical appearance. In fact, for some men appearance and function were better post-operatively because the discomfort of the previously enlarged testis was relieved.

You're All Right, the Left One's Still There

Details of relative or actual frequency of sexual activity were not raised by the men during interviews, and so no comment can be made because the men themselves did not talk about this. The issues they did raise in connection with sexual functioning were linked to whether or not they had a partner, whether they had been given any information about sexual functioning, and whether sexual activity was or was not a problem for them.

Two men were single and not in sexual relationships at the time of interview, but did wonder how things would work out if they did get into a relationship. P14 said:

I think the only other scenario that would affect me was if I was – erm – having a sexual relationship with a girl . . . But then if you were having a sexual relationship with a girl and you were into that kind of intimacy they really must care about you enough not to care that you've only got one, if you see what I mean.

Three other men who did have partners reported that loss of the testis and sexual relations were not a problem for either side of the couple. The remaining men made no mention of this aspect.

One of the most striking features of this interview theme was the number who said that they had not been given any information about sexual functioning by medical staff, or that they had had to gain information by direct questioning. Information from doctors tended to have been given in euphemistic terms such as 'You can lead a perfectly normal life', and only two men felt that they had been 'told everything' without having to ask. P11 had particular praise for his surgeon, and this seemed to be related to the fact that he provided information throughout their association.

Direct questioning of doctors by the men seemed to be unusual, but for P2 this had been important:

The first thing I asked him was, 'Does it alter your sex life?', you know. And he said, 'No.' And he said, 'I had one done 18 years ago', and he said, 'No'.

This man supposed that:

the first question that every consultant gets asked as soon as he tells somebody who's going to lose their testicle is – er – will we still get our sex life?

But this supposition seemed incorrect and most men had neither been given nor felt able to seek information on this point. One man who could not remember being given information about sexual function by doctors had sought this from a nurse, but he was the only one to mention nurses as a source of information.

Another man had not had any information about sexual functioning until it was mentioned briefly at the hospital where he went for sperm banking prior to chemotherapy. But he explained that while he was ill he was not really thinking about how this would be affected and such ideas were 'very low on your list of priorities' and fell well behind 'getting back to health, and your life back into order'.

In the face of lack of information from professionals, some men used other sources. P14 was informed by the surgeon that he 'would not be affected in any way' but had sought clarification from a medical student friend who was able to provide more detailed information. Another man gained information from a friend who had also had testicular cancer and seemed to have been given much more information.

Men's descriptions of their sexual functioning and how they felt about this could be divided into three categories as follows:

- Poor, deteriorating or no function: problem.
- Poor, deteriorating or no function: not a problem.
- Good, 'normal' or improved function: not a problem.

These three states did not appear to be discrete and the men might move between them at different times.

Poor or absent functioning

Poor or absent functioning which was a problem affected three men for whom enlargement pre-operatively had impeded sexual activity. One likened the testicle to 'a big tennis ball' between his legs, while another commented that the effects of the swelling on his sexual relationship had been both physical and psychological (P7):

> I live with my girlfriend, and it's just started to affect me – you know – sex relationship. I wasn't as good as I used to be. Prior to that, over the years, like I say, it swells and goes down, goes away, but over the years it never affected me that way. But over the last few months things were getting a bit serious down there, you know . . . I think it was a combination of both, really. It was psychological and I think it was physical as well.

For another man sexual function after the operation was described as problematic and he explained the situation in this way (P2):

> I put it down to the long emotional strain on both of us; that we'd been emotionally on a tightrope, really. Although – you know – having said that we sailed through it all; it's still there, and I put it down to prolonged

emotional experience of 2 to 3 months, which it has been now from the start up to the present day, of emotions being up and down, up and down. Very torn. I put it down to that.

However, by the time of his third interview this disquiet was no longer evident (P2):

> . . . it's never bothered me. That's – you know – once, once we'd established that we could still, you know, have sex – then we didn't have any problems.

It may be that he had forgotten the past difficulties or that events had taken on a different perspective with time.

Others with poor or absent sexual functioning did not see this as problematic and one said that sex had been 'put on the back burner'. Five of these men were receiving chemotherapy at the time and the major reason they gave was that they were tired as a result of treatment. They viewed this situation as temporary and so were not unduly concerned.

Two men talked about priorities and how other aspects of their relationships with their wives were far more important (P1):

> It's been different from normal because we still sort of kiss but nothing more than that.

His wife was present at the interview and added:

> Well, there's no sexual side to it, but I mean, it's not really affected us emotionally – I think it's because we can talk.

Another man described how he differentiates between sexual activity and expressions of love for his wife, saying (P10):

> You can actually split it between actual sex life and love life. Because the affection I've had off the wife is fantastic, the support she's given me. There's the affection, you know. The affection's still there for both of us, but the actual sex life is put on the back burner, kind of thing.

Some men reported that their sex lives were normal and that there was no problem. The most striking thing about their descriptions was their brevity, giving an impression that they did not want this topic to be probed. The reasons for such brief answers may be many and varied. It could be that they were more concerned about sexual functioning than they felt able, willing or indeed had the necessary language to express. The interviewer's presence will have influenced what they were prepared to say, whether they felt able to disclose their thoughts, and whether they were responding to what they thought she wanted to hear. On one hand, she was a stranger and a female and was asking about a possible taboo subject in our culture. On the other hand, they knew that she was a nurse, and it is culturally acceptable for a female nurse to ask for intimate information from a male patient.

In summary, in relation to sexual functioning lack of information again emerges as a crucial issue. For many couples, physical sexual activity was less important than the emotional side of their relationships and this support had meant a great deal to the men at this difficult time in their lives. Some men experienced sexual difficulties due to the tiredness resulting from chemo-therapy. For others, orchidectomy had improved their sex lives because the awkward swelling had now gone. However, some men did not seem able to talk to the interviewer about sexual functioning, probably because of cultural norms about discussing intimate topics with strangers of the opposite sex and/or the difficulty that men in our culture may have about speaking openly about their emotions.

Kids are About the Last Thing on My Mind at the Moment

Fertility was an issue for men who had no children or who might want to add to their families in the future. Eight men came into this category, with three being childless at the time, two already having children with a previous partner, and three already having children with their present partners. The remaining 10 men said either that they did not want more children or were not concerned about future fertility, and three of these were currently childless. Seven of these considered their families to be complete and two had had vasectomies. The overall impression was that at this time fertility was not a major concern, and that foremost in men's minds was the fact that they had cancer and, for some, coping with chemotherapy and its side-effects.

Evidence that fertility was a lesser consideration for some men comes from the fact that some men chose not to delay further treatment in order to take up an offer of sperm banking (P18):

> [The doctor] started to explain to me about radiotherapy – 'Do you want to store any sperm?' I said, 'Well, no, I'd rather just get on with it' . . . So forget storing sperm if it means – because I think there's a 3-week wait with that, isn't it? They take some over a number of weeks, don't they . . . Yeah, well, I thought, well I – I don't want to wait that long. I just wanted to get on with it.

Two men who expressed very positive desires for more children both took the decision not to delay treatment in order to bank sperm, believing that it was important to have treatment as early as possible. In practice it is rarely so vital that a short delay to allow sperm banking would be prejudicial. Also sperm banking is usually offered to men being treated with chemotherapy and not for radiotherapy.

Another man who wanted more children was pressed by his wife not to delay treatment for sperm banking. However, in this case the doctor intervened:

> [My wife] was saying things straight away, and I think, em, Dr X realised that and said, 'No, just slow down. It's something you've got to discuss,

you know; you just can't go "snap" and make a decision . . .' We talked about it in considerable length and we decided to go and deposit some sperm.

The youngest man, however, who was a 20-year-old single man, showed his deep concern when talking about how he would feel if the cancer spread and he had to have a second orchidectomy (P14):

. . . If it happened again that would be a big thing. If it happened on the other one, and I had to have the other one taken off me . . . Well, that would be – that would probably be quite devastating because (a) I wouldn't be able to have children and (b) – you know – it's – it gets rid of – erm – I'd feel at lot – em – a lot less likely to want to have sex with anybody, I think.

He went on to explain his feelings in this way:

Yeah, not so much body image for me. More I wouldn't be able to have children, I think . . . Because that's – your whole – it's like your whole self being taken away then. You're just a person then. You're not a person with the potential to be – other people through your children. Do you see what I mean?

Another single man with no children spoke of another difficulty he had encountered. He felt that he had been provided with little information about fertility-related matters and was not offered sperm banking. He considered that the doctor had stereotyped him as homosexual on the basis of being single at the age of 38 and being 'in show business'. He stated that (P3):

The only one thing what ever annoyed me – and it didn't dramatically annoy me – but I was – D asked, and I was asked twice in [X hospital] by doctors – and that was my status in life – that I was single. And they asked if I was homosexual . . . And on the third time I just happened to turn and said, 'Well, why are you asking this?' . . . 'Is it just because the age I am and I'm not married? Is it that?' And he said, 'Oh, well, we've got to ask these questions'.

He returned to this issue in the second interview and was obviously still feeling angry about what had happened:

I would have liked to have turned round – they see that you're a novice, you see, because you're frightened – well, you're not frightened, but you're bothered. I'd like to have turned round to the doctors . . . I'd like to have turned round and said, 'Mind your own bloody business!' . . . But you don't – you don't. You see, you do not. Because you submit to people in white coats – you know, the doctor.

This man was angry about what he perceived to be an unwanted intrusion into his private life and assumptions made about his life-style based on superficial information, and he felt powerless to answer as he wanted to because he was in a dependent position.

In the main, then, fertility took second place to cancer and its treatment for the majority of men, including one who had first been found to have a problem through attendance at a fertility clinic. However, for very young men the position is likely to be more ambiguous, as exemplified by the youngest man interviewed for whom the symbolic significance of fertility seemed an important issue. Additionally, on this theme as well as the others discussed, lack of information and misunderstanding were features of some men's accounts.

Issues for Nurses

Young men with testicular cancer will probably have their first contact with nurses in a district general hospital while having their orchidectomy. Usually, their stay in hospital will be very brief because of the minor physical nature of the operation and because they are generally young and otherwise healthy. Nurses working on these wards will not encounter many instances of testicular cancer, but it is important for them to have knowledge of the condition, its treatment and the possible implications of this in order to meet these patients' needs.

Lack of information, misinformation and misunderstandings seemed common among the men interviewed, and nurses did not feature in their stories to any great extent. This suggests that opportunities to provide information and support are being missed, which may be even more important when the in-patient period is so short. Advantage should be taken of every opportunity to assess the man's knowledge and worries, as well as those of his partner or close supporters if appropriate.

A thorough nursing assessment is essential, and nurses should be particularly alert to issues of sexuality which may arise. The assessment should be conducted in private and a sensitive, non-judgmental climate should be promoted to encourage the man to express any concerns. It is quite likely that nurses in this situation will not be able to answer specific or specialised questions, but it is important to pick up cues to problems and make a referral to someone who is able to respond.

Following orchidectomy men are referred to a specialist cancer centre and their main contact is likely to be with doctors. Some will undergo a short course of radiotherapy as an out-patient, again with little if any nursing input. The main and continuing contact for all men will be the out-patient clinic, where monitoring for recurrence is undertaken. Out-patient clinics are invariably very busy, providing little time for talking, and again minimal contact with nurses.

The study discussed in this chapter was a small one, based at one specialist centre, and therefore it is not possible to generalise findings and make claims about other men's likely experiences. However, lack of information is a recurrent cause of dissatisfaction among patients and poor communication is the second most common complaint to the Health Ombudsman (Health Service Commissioner 1993).

When a patient's problems are related to such a personal and vital topic as sexuality, it is both particularly important that their concerns are addressed and more likely that they may not be. Staff – doctor and nurses alike – may not have been trained in inter-personal skills and counselling and may therefore inadvertently miss clues given out by patients about their needs (Stewart, McWhinney and Buck 1979, Bond 1982, Maguire 1985). If the experiences of men interviewed in this study are typical, then a 'Clinical Nurse Specialist' approach may be appropriate. The role of breast nurse specialists has been developed since we have become aware of their potential for detecting and minimising physical and psychological complications and assisting social recovery (Maguire et al 1983). It would be valuable to introduce a similar nursing service for men experiencing testicular cancer and to evaluate outcome from the point of view of patient satisfaction and cost-effectiveness in the same way as has been done with other Clinical Nurse Specialist roles (Graveley & Littlefield 1992).

In the meantime, nurses having contact with these men, particularly in the early stages of diagnosis and treatment in general practices and district general hospitals, need to be able to carry out an appropriate nursing assessment and plan and deliver care which responds to their needs, particularly for information and emotional support.

Assessment

As well as conducting the usual nursing assessment, the kinds of areas to explore include:

- whether or not the man has a sexual partner or close support person, his views of this relationship, and the type and extent of emotional support available to him;
- what he understands about his diagnosis and treatment and how these may affect his body image, self-concept, fertility, sexual functioning and relationships;
- how he feels about these matters, and whether he has any major concerns or worries;
- what he knows about measures to ameliorate these effects, for example counselling, sperm banking;
- how he usually copes with stressful life events;
- how he is currently coping with actual or potential diagnosis of cancer, and any other current significant life events.

Problems/Needs Identification

Following the assessment, problems or needs identified may include:

- fear and uncertainty concerning the actual or potential diagnosis of cancer and its implications;
- lack of knowledge about testicular cancer, its prognosis, treatment, effects and implications;
- lack of knowledge/concern about loss of the testis and its implications;
- lack of knowledge/concern about potential effects on sexual functioning;
- lack of knowledge/concern about potential effects on fertility, and measures to maximise possibilities of having children in the future.

Setting Goals

The major goal for the man himself is likely to be that he will be cured and suffer no complications. Other goals may include:

- minimising fear and anxiety;
- maximising knowledge about and control over the situation;
- maintaining self-esteem, self-concept and body image;
- minimising sexual dysfunction;
- maximising ability to have children, if desired.

Nursing Interventions

Nursing assessment provides the first opportunity for intervention, as already discussed, by providing an opportunity for the man and his partner or other support person(s) to communicate their information and support needs and other concerns within a sympathetic environment. Depending on what is learned and communicated within the assessment, further interventions may focus on the following.

- Providing – or ensuring that others provide – accurate information about surgery, further treatment (chemotherapy/radiotherapy), possible side-effects, complications and outcomes, prognosis and future treatment and monitoring.
- Providing care and support through the surgical experience, with particular attention to anxiety and fear
- Providing information and referral if appropriate for specialist care or services such as:
  sperm banking
  prosthetic testis implant
  specialist/psychosexual counselling.

- Encouraging men and their partners/support persons to talk openly and freely about the treatment process, their reactions and feelings, and to ask for help if they would like this.
- Maintaining open communication with other health professionals in an attempt to discover/minimise contradictory and inconsistent information-giving.

Nurses working in general practice and out-patient clinic settings, as well as those in surgical wards, need to be aware of all these issues, to be alert for cues to undetected problems or unmet needs, and to give care or make referrals to other professionals in this way. Men with testicular cancer are extremely likely to be cured of their disease, but they may have very real sexuality-related needs at any stage in the treatment process and for some time afterwards. It is vital that the real successes of medical management of these men are matched by care and assistance in coping with the experience.

Acknowledgements

The study on which this chapter is based was generously funded by the Cancer Relief Macmillan Fund, and we are grateful for their support.

References

Blackmore C (1988) The impact of orchidectomy upon the sexuality of the man with testicular cancer. *Cancer Nursing,* **11**, 1, 33–40.

Blandy J P, Hope-Stone H F and Dayan A D (1970) *Tumours of the Testicle.* London: William Heinemann.

Bond S (1982) Communications in cancer nursing. In Cahoon M C (ed.) *Recent Advances in Nursing 3. Cancer Nursing,* Ch. 1. Edinburgh: Churchill Livingstone.

Cassileth B R and Steinfeld A D (1987) Psychological preparation of the patient and family. *Cancer,* **60**, 3 (Supplement), 547–552.

Cooper A (1982) Disabilities and how to live with them: Hodgkin's disease. *Lancet,* **i**, 8272, 612–613.

Douchez J, Droz J P, Desclaux B, Allain Y, Fargeot P, Caty A and Charrot P (1993) Quality of life in long-term survivors of nonseminomatous germ cell testicular tumours. *Journal of Urology,* **149**, 3, 498–501.

Graveley E A and Littlefield J H (1992) A cost-effective analysis of three staffing models for the delivery of low-risk prenatal care. *American Journal of Public Health,* **82**, 2, 180–184.

Hannah M T, Gritz E R, Wellisch D K, Forbair P, Hoppe R T, Bloom J R, Sun G-W, Varghese A, Cosgrove M and Spiegel D (1992) Changes in marital and sexual functioning in long-term survivors and their spouses: testicular cancer versus Hodgkin's disease. *Psycho-Oncology,* **1**, 89–103.

Health Service Commissioner (1993) *Annual Report for 1992–1993,* 764. London: HMSO.

Hendry W E, Stedronska J, Jones C R, Blackmore C A, Barrett A and Peckham M J (1983) Semen analysis in testicular cancer and Hodgkin's disease: pre- and post-treatment findings and implications for cryopreservation. *British Journal of Urology*, **55**, 6, 769–773.

Horwich A (ed.) (1991) *Testicular Cancer: Investigation and Management*. London: Chapman & Hall Medical.

Kaasa S, Aass N, Mastekaasa A, Lund E and Fossa S D (1991) Psychosocial well-being in testicular cancer patients. *European Journal of Cancer*, **27**, 9, 1091–1095.

Kennedy B J, Tellegen A, Kennedy S and Havernick N (1976) Psychological response of patients cured of advanced cancer. *Cancer*, **38**, 5, 2184–2191.

Loescher L J, Clark L, Atwood J R, Leigh S and Lamb G (1990) The impact of the cancer experience on long-term survivors. *Oncology Nursing Forum*, **17**, 2, 223–229.

Maguire P (1985) Deficiencies in key interpersonal skills. In Kagan C M (ed.) *Interpersonal Skills in Nursing: Research and Applications*, Ch. 8. London: Chapman & Hall.

Maguire P, Brooke M, Tait A, Thomas C and Sellwood R (1983) The effect of counselling on physical disability and social recovery after mastectomy. *Clinical Oncology*, **9**, 319–324.

Moynihan C (1987) Testicular cancer: the psychosocial problems of patients and their relatives. *Cancer Surveys*, **6**, 3, 477–510.

Office of Population Censuses and Surveys (1985) *Cancer Statistics (Registration) England and Wales, Series MB1*, No. 18. London: HMSO.

Peckham M J (1988) Testicular cancer. *Acta Oncologica*, **27**, 4, 439–453.

Pike M C, Chilvers C and Peckham M J (1986) Effect of age at orchidopexy on risk of testicular cancer. *Lancet*, **i**, 1246–1248.

Rieker P P, Edbril S D and Garnick M B (1985) Curative testis cancer therapy: psychosocial sequelae. *Journal of Clinical Oncology*, **3**, 8, 1117–1126.

Senturia Y D (1987) The epidemiology of testicular cancer. *Cancer Topics*, **6**, 9, 102–104.

Stewart M A, McWhinney I R and Buck C W (1979) The doctor–patient relationship and its effect on outcome. *Journal of the Royal College of General Practitioners*, **29**, 77–82.

Stuart N S A, Grundy R, Woodroffe C M & Cullen M H (1990) Quality of life after treatment for testicular cancer – the patient's view. *European Journal of Cancer*, **26**, 3, 291–294.

Chapter 4
Bad Women and Good Customers: Scapegoating, Female Prostitution and HIV
Jean Faugier

Introduction

In 1990 the World Health Organization dedicated World AIDS Day and the events surrounding it to the issue of women and AIDS. Four years on, the problems posed by HIV for women have reached even greater and more worrying proportions. It is estimated that, of the total current cases of AIDS, at least one-third are women and that by the year 2000 there will be equal numbers of men and women with AIDS (World Health Organization 1992). Chin (1990) points out that the vast majority of these women will have contracted the virus through unprotected (by use of a condom) heterosexual intercourse, which is globally the major route of transmission for HIV.

It has taken some time for policy-makers and leaders of the medical profession to recognise the personal, social and economic impact of HIV/AIDS upon women, and the long-term effect that this will have on society. However, up to now the influence of women at policy level and in determining service provision has been minimal, and AIDS in women often still tends to be overlooked. This is due, in the main, to the still relatively small percentage of AIDS cases among women in Britain and other European countries, although in Africa tens of thousands of women are suffering from AIDS and many more are infected with HIV. Another area of real concern is the fact that relatively little research has been done on the pattern of HIV infection in women; indeed, most research has been undertaken on samples of gay men or drug users who are predominantly white and male, and women who turn up for treatment presenting with HIV-related symptoms come up against medical and nursing staff who have formed their impression of AIDS from a male-dominated model and have very little knowledge of the clinical manifestations of AIDS/HIV among women, which frequently differ significantly from those described in research on men (Richardson 1989).

A growing number of AIDS activists are now attempting to get the Centre for Disease Control to broaden its definition of AIDS in line with the point made by Elbaz (1993, 801) that

The current definition excludes whole communities of individuals who do not fit the conventional criteria. Women and injecting drug users, in particular, are excluded from the official definition because the opportunistic infections they contract are specific to their physiology and environment. Consequently those populations are excluded from research, healthcare and social services supported by AIDS funding.

Heterosexual AIDS

Of particular significance for women is the tendency of the media and whole layers of the establishment to attempt to play down the possibility of heterosexual transmission of HIV outside the continent of Africa. The association of women with the spread of sexually transmitted diseases is one which is constant throughout history: 'certain kinds of women' are seen as a reservoir of infection, a temptation which will befall honourable men and one to be avoided at all costs. Sontag (1991) points out that, like cancer, AIDS is a fatal disease which produces the feelings of shame previously linked to cancer, and also carries with it the fact that the answer to 'why me?' is not obscure. AIDS is not a mysterious affliction appearing to strike at random. Sontag clearly states that this is a disease which reveals the person suffering from it to be a member of a particular group, a risk group, easily identifiable by everyone – parents, friends, neighbours and colleagues.

At the beginning of the epidemic, particularly in the United States and Western Europe, homosexual men were the first people to be affected by HIV and AIDS, closely followed by injecting drug users, who are predominantly male. To be infected with HIV and to develop AIDS is therefore seen very much as a stigmatised condition. In the words of Goffman (1968), it confers upon the sufferer a 'spoiled identity'. Indeed, in many cases, the people affected by AIDS have a dual 'spoiled identity': not only do they have a disease which carries tremendous stigma, but one which frequently strips away defences from another identity already connected with very strong social stigmas. This is particularly true in the case of gay men, injecting drug users and, of course, prostitutes. Again, Sontag very lucidly points to the persistent belief that illness both reveals and punishes some sort of moral laxity; in other words, the disease is seen as the end result of a life that is full of blame and the AIDS sufferer is declared to be guilty as a result of his/her previous lifestyle. The strong contrast between the terminology used to describe gay men, drug users and prostitutes, as opposed to people who have contracted AIDS through blood products or transfusions, provides a lucid example of the apportioning of such blame: haemophiliacs and children are described as the 'innocent' victims of the AIDS epidemic, which clearly places all the other groups in the guilty category.

The association of female prostitution with sexually transmitted diseases and drug misuse is certainly not a new development. Plant (1990) points to the well-known historical links between sexually transmitted disease and women using drugs, including alcohol; neither is this view of female prostitutes as responsible for infection confined to the past: a number of medical practitioners, including Robertson (1987), a GP well known for his innovative work with drug users, continue to refer to female prostitutes as 'a reservoir of infection'. As Darrow (1984) describes, studies from a number of centres confirm that female prostitutes do have higher rates of sexually transmitted diseases than those obtaining for the general population, hence the perception that they pose a major public health threat, which has in turn resulted in making them scapegoats for the AIDS epidemic. The important players in the heterosexual transmission of HIV/AIDS are then seen as 'loose' or 'bad' women rather than any particular responsibility being ascribed to heterosexual men.

The available data on the association between prostitution and the spread of the HIV epidemic is unclear and certainly different in terms of geographical location. Padian (1988) shows that prostitution in sub-Saharan Africa has clearly played a very significant part in the continued epidemic amongst heterosexuals. Similarly, studies of prostitutes in Kenya have shown that some of the high rates of transmission from prostitutes may be explained by a higher incidence of significant co-factors, particularly genital ulceration. Suggestions that non-circumcision in men and the use of oral contraceptives by women may influence the transmission of the virus have also been made in relation to African prostitution (International Conference on AIDS 1992).

In Europe and the United States, the association between non-drug-using female prostitutes and HIV infection is low and currently does not seem to be playing a major part in HIV transmission. Prostitution is only significantly linked to the transmission of HIV in Europe and the United States when drug use is involved. As Nichols (1989, 30) states,

> The geographic distribution of HIV infection among heterosexual adults and adolescents with no known risk factors parallels the geographic distribution of AIDS cases among intravenous drug users and is highest in the New York City area and Puerto Rico, moderately high elsewhere on the east coast and in California, and below five per cent in other areas of the country.

High rates of HIV in European prostitutes also appear to be linked to drug injecting, either in themselves or their partners. Goldberg et al (1988), Tirelli, Rezza and Guillani (1989) and Doerr et al (1990) all identified higher levels of HIV infection among drug-injecting prostitutes than non-injecting prostitutes.

AIDS in the UK

Following both speculation from the media and epidemiological evidence of increased heterosexual transmission of HIV, a small number of studies into

HIV risk behaviour and prostitutes were funded from a variety of sources in several areas within the UK. While the research methodologies employed by these studies differ widely, they nevertheless provide a baseline of important information relating to possible risk behaviour among prostitutes and their clients.

In a study of Birmingham prostitutes, Kinnel (1989) employed a structured interview schedule administered by current and former prostitutes. Two hundred and fifty-eight interviews were conducted, and no major difference was found between drug injectors (15 per cent of the sample) and non-drug users. Of particular interest was the finding that drug injectors were less likely to be working the streets than non-drug-using women, and were more likely to work in saunas or off-street premises. Furthermore, the study reported that the frequency of high-risk sexual activity was greater as was the rate of pay in 'off-street' working, findings which differ from all subsequent studies.

A study employing very similar methodology was undertaken by Morgan Thomas (1990) in Edinburgh in which 103 female prostitutes were contacted and data were collected by the use of a standardised questionnaire. Approximately 28 per cent of the sample were injecting drug users and 8 per cent of the entire sample reported rarely or never using condoms with clients.

In a cohort study of genito-urinary medicine clinic attenders in London, Ward and Day (1990) investigated the risk behaviour of 100 female prostitutes who were then followed up at clinic attendances over a period of two years. Only 19 per cent of the sample worked predominantly as street prostitutes, and only 7.4 per cent were injecting drug users. Condom use with clients was found to be as high as 96 per cent, while condom use with other sexual partners was only 17.6 per cent. Three of the women were found to be HIV sero-positive, two of whom had shared injecting equipment and one who seemed to have been infected by her sero-positive drug-using boyfriend.

Work of a different methodological nature was undertaken by McKeganey and Barnard (1992). In a qualitative study employing ethnographic methodo logy, 208 female prostitutes were contacted in the red light area of Glasgow and short contact interviews and field notes were the major means of data collection. In addition, the researchers undertook to provide a service by delivery of condoms and clean injecting equipment to women working in that area. Although the researchers experienced very little difficulty in interviewing women about drug use, they readily acknowledge the problems they had in engaging women on the topic of sex in a very short, 10–15-minute interview in the work situation. Obviously, in such circumstances, distractions from possible clients and, more importantly, peer pressure from other women, make openness about sexual risk behaviour difficult, not to say unlikely.

Scapegoating

Weeks (1989) points to three distinct phases in the social response to AIDS up to the present time. He refers to the 'dawning crisis' from 1981 to 1982, the 'moral panic' from 1982 to 1985 and 'crisis management' from 1985 onwards. From the very beginning, of course, gay men in particular have been at the receiving end of much of the prejudice and scapegoating that has been induced by the media. However, when it became apparent that the epidemic was not going to be confined to socially marginalised groups, such as gay men, drug users and female prostitutes, but was also being heterosexually transmitted to the wider population, a more appropriate scapegoat than gay men had to be found. Scrambler et al (1990) point out that female prostitutes fitted the bill very nicely for this role, and that they proved particularly useful as scapegoats for the spread of the epidemic in Africa. However, this also applies to the United Kingdom, the United States and other Western European countries, where the association of prostitution with the spread of AIDS continues to hold sway even in the light of very little research evidence, thus allowing those with certain political agendas to attack women from yet another angle and particularly, of course, to concentrate their attacks on women who are economically deprived.

There are historical precedents for this attack on women who are seen as sexually bad and in particular women who prostitute. The Contagious Diseases Acts of 1864, 1866 and 1869 defined venereal diseases as transmitted by women and made no attempt whatsoever to restrain men from placing themselves at risk. What the Acts did do was to provide the police and the criminal justice system with the power to force female prostitutes into medical quarantine. Pateman (1988, 264) quotes the report of the Royal Commission into the Acts which states that

> There is no comparison to be made between prostitutes and the men who consort with them. With the one sex, the offence is committed as a matter of gain; with the other, it is an irregular indulgence of a natural impulse.

Attitudes to Sexuality

Such a double standard approach to the sexuality of men and women is, of course, quite common and has had a serious effect on campaigns to encourage young women to take a more active role in relation to their sexual health and sexuality. The relationship of sex, gender and power has meant that many young women find it impossible to anticipate sex: to carry a condom is seen as proof of looseness and also as undermining the essential degree of trust which they are brought up to believe must exist in loving heterosexual relationships (Holland et al 1990, Araldsen and Hansen 1993). However, in contrast with African countries, the West is characterised by relatively low rates of HIV infection among prostitutes unless those prostitutes are also drug users themselves or have partners who inject drugs. The Center for Disease Control in Atlanta, USA, estimates that the infection rate of IV drug-using prostitutes in the USA is at least four times higher than that found in non-IV drug-using prostitutes (Center for Disease Control 1992).

In the process of becoming 'civilised', sexual aspects of life have also become privatised. However, unlike other private bodily functions with which nursing is concerned, acts defined as sexual (the experience and perception of other people as sexual beings) are social constructions built around the biological differences between male and female. Sexual aspects of social life are complex inasmuch as:

1. They are integral to the relations between men and women.
2. They are products of the inter-relationships between biology and culture.

HIV raises a whole range of very troublesome issues for women, focusing around the areas of risk and trust, sexual pressures, the concept of romantic love and all the other aspects seen as crucial to the development of relationships between the sexes. Anxiety about sexually transmitted disease is difficult to insert into this scenario because it immediately brings into play the notions of intimacy, love and trust. Many young women lack confidence and self-esteem and automatically assume that men are much more competent actors in terms of sex. The whole area of negotiation of safer sex is a complex and dangerous one, fraught with many serious difficulties. For most young women, the use of condoms poses an embarrassment problem at every single stage, from buying them to carrying them and requesting their use (Holland et al 1990). Until such issues are no longer at odds with what our society believes to be a 'feminine identity' and until women are no longer brought up to assume that they are to be swept off their feet, that sex is simply something which is to happen to them, and that they are merely the victims of male desire, they will continue to be at serious risk of HIV. In a qualitative study of 50 women who had contracted HIV through heterosexual sex with a steady partner, Verrisimo, Pucheu and Morais (1993, 808) report that:

> The self image constructed by these women was characterised by low self-esteem, emotional and sexual passiveness, subjectiveness before others' desires, emotional dependence and self-confidence limitation despite their active behaviour in other aspects of their lives.

Working through these contradictions is not easy, as the sexual empowerment of women implies a direct threat to male power. In this sense, HIV raises the whole range of gender relations issues. Giving young women sexual empowerment also contradicts the messages of abstinence, monogamy and marriage coming from the establishment; these are compromised messages for most women of all ages. Young women in particular will find it very difficult to talk openly about previous sexual relationships when they are not supposed to have had any, since they are expected to come to the relationship of their life without any experience and possibly even in a virginal state.

Any sexual health education in nursing implies coming to terms and dealing with the identity of the client. Many female drug users with whom I have been working over the past two years are damaged, sexually abused young women, and find it extremely difficult to exert power in sexual relationships – even, for that matter, in prostitution. The idea that women who work as prostitutes fall into the 'tart with a heart' category or that they are older, self-assured women who know exactly what they are doing is a total and dangerous myth. In actual fact, prostitution involves a high level of damage, violence and a very worrying lack of expertise and skill in sexual terms.

The Manchester Study

In my own study examining the risk behaviour of drug-using and non-drug-using female prostitutes and their clients, 150 women working as prostitutes in the Manchester area were interviewed. Fifty were non-drug users and 100 were drug users. In the main, respondents were recruited to the study by direct outreach work, either in the streets or at court. The majority of the sample (56 per cent) were between 18 and 25 years of age at the time of interview. However, 19 per cent of the sample were over 30, and five women over 40. The oldest respondent was 47 years old and the youngest 15. The drug users tended to predominate in the younger age groups: 35 per cent of drug users were under 21 as opposed to 26 per cent of non-users, the figures rising to 69 per cent and 58 per cent, respectively, for the under-25 age group.

A significant number of the women (47 per cent) had had disrupted schooling: they had, in fact, failed to remain at school until the statutory school-leaving age although, for a small number of older women in the sample, a lower statutory age would have applied. Just over half the sample (53 per cent) did complete schooling, with only 2 per cent remaining at school longer than the time required by law. Again the drug-using women were more likely than their non-drug-using counterparts to have suffered disrupted or incomplete schooling.

The vast majority of respondents lived in rented accommodation owned by private landlords, or in a minority of cases by the Local Authority. A significant group of younger, more vulnerable drug-using women were technically homeless, living either in a squat or sleeping on a friend's floor. Many of these women frequently found themselves engaged in a sexual relationship in order to secure accommodation. One young woman interviewed was typical of this group: she was 17 years old, pregnant and living in a squat with six male injecting drug-users and a pit bull terrier. Homelessness has been cited in a number of studies as predictive of high-risk behaviour among injecting drug users (Marmor et al 1987; Hartgers 1989; Klee et al 1990).

Drug-using women were significantly more likely to have been placed in care as children. Although questions relating to previous sexual abuse were considered inappropriate in a research interview without any supportive follow-up, none the less a number of women volunteered such information, as illustrated by the following quotations from interviews.

Jane, aged 25, drug user
When I was 13, I put myself into care. I went to the social and asked to be taken into care. My mother was an alcoholic out drinking every night and

I was left at home with me dad. He was sexually assaulting me from when I was about ten. I never told the social workers that, I said I had been raped when a man broke in when they were both out drinking, but I think they knew what was going on. I didn't want to go back there, so they put me in a home.

Yvonne, aged 21, drug user
I went in care before I left school, so I haven't had much schooling, like, after I was 14. I was always running away 'cause there was this pervert at the first home who kept messing about with me every time he was on at night, so eventually they put me in a lock-up run by nuns.

Pauline, aged 21, drug user
I were on the run from this children's home and I knew this guy. I had stayed at his house before 'cause he knew a lad I used to go out with. He gave me a few cans of Special Brew and he must have dropped some pills in 'em 'cause he raped me anally and all I can remember is the pain and the bedroom going round.

As might be imagined, due to the need to feed considerable drug habits, the drug-using women were forced to work longer hours and more nights per week than the non-drug-using prostitutes. This frequently involved working in isolated situations and in appalling weather conditions.

Mary, aged 23, drug user
I work seven nights a week and God knows how many hours I am out there sometimes. I have been picked up by the police at 5 a.m. and I would have been stood there from 1 a.m. 'cause I used to go out, make some money, then go home for a dig (injection), and then come back out and make some more money for the morning, kind of thing. So I could go out at 7 p.m., go home twice for a dig, and still be out at 5 a.m.

This need to work more frequently resulted in the drug users having significantly more clients per week than non-drug-using women. Seventy per cent of drug users reported more than 30 clients per week as opposed to 30 per cent of non-users. Sexual services provided by the women ranged from simple masturbation (hand relief) to quite complex sado-masochistic activities and role-play situations. However, by far the most common service requested by clients was penetrative vaginal intercourse. Although many of the women from both groups would suggest during the interview that they attempted whenever possible to restrict clients to non-penetrative activities such as hand relief, the data on what sexual activities they were in fact performing present a rather different story: only 3 per cent of drug users and 18 per cent of non-users gave hand relief as their most frequent sexual service. Penetrative sexual activity was very high for both groups, with 50 per cent of drug users and 58 per cent of non-users saying that this was their most frequent activity. This figure refers, in the majority of cases, to vaginal sex, but 3 per cent of drug users and 8 per cent of non-users did also report offering anal sex. However, anal sex was not the most frequently offered service in any individual case. Interestingly, when pressed to offer more expensive services in order to obtain funds for their habit, drug-using women were more likely (21 per cent) to offer a combination of oral stimulation followed by penetrative sex than were non-drug-using women (4 per cent).

The majority of respondents reported insisting on condom use with clients at all times. Many women were aware of the other infections, in addition to HIV, that they were leaving themselves open to if they failed to do so. However, a very significant number of drug-using women (33 per cent) and 12 per cent of non-drug using women were, under certain circumstances, prepared to dispense with the use of condoms. For the drug users, the motivation was very clear and stemmed from a simple desperation to get sufficient money in as short a time as possible. These women described scenarios in which they had been offered more money, sometimes not that much more, for unprotected sex, and had dispensed with condoms so that they could leave the beat immediately in order to buy drugs.

Sharon, aged 21, drug user

It's the crack, you see, it's all you think about. It makes you go to lengths that you would not have done before, like doing punters without a Durex. You don't think about it till afterwards, especially with all this AIDS stuff and everything . . . but at the time, you just don't think about that. There have been times when I've had no Durex and I've walked past the van (outreach service) where you can get them for nothing, but I am so wired up I have to go, no time to stop for Durex, I just want the next punter for the next 25 pounds so I can fuck off.

The motivations of the non-drug-users were also financial although, in all but one case, the choice of client whom they would allow to dispense with condoms depended on how long the prostitute had known him. These women were prepared to dispense with condoms for more money when they felt they knew the client sufficiently to ascertain the risk to themselves from doing so. Frequently, such assessments were based on very superficial judgements of issues such as cleanliness, reliability and kindness, and owed little to any real understanding of the client's life.

Sheila, aged 25, non-drug user

Well, he's been coming to me for about five years now, regular as clockwork every two weeks. He's a salesman from out of town. I am pretty sure he only sees me. I mean, once or twice he's rung and I have not been able to see him and he says he didn't go to any other girl. Well, I mean, he's only here for 2 hours, he pays 70 quid and he brings me a bottle of Tia Maria as well.

However, the most important players in relation to unprotected sexual activity in prostitution are obviously the men who repeatedly request it. Almost all respondents to the study reported being asked at some time to perform unprotected vaginal or oral sex. Sixty per cent of the entire sample claimed that such requests were a daily occurrence. Drug users were significantly more likely to report such requests, and it is difficult to ascertain to what extent this may be due to their longer hours on the streets or the fact that they may be known by punters as women who might be prepared to deliver such services under certain circumstances.

The majority of respondents had a regular male sexual partner and were living with one at the time of interview. This divided up into 62 per cent for drug-using women and 72 per cent for non-drug users. Predictably, the drug users were significantly more likely to have an injecting drug user as a sexual partner (42 per cent) than the non-users (8 per cent). However, there was no particular difference between the two groups in terms of condom use with regular partners: 57 out of the 62 drug users with a partner never used condoms with them, as was the case for 32 of the 36 non-drug-using women. They explained this behaviour in the following ways.

Vera, aged 30, drug user
Why use condoms with me fella? No way, he would kill me. I wouldn't dream of suggesting it, not with him.

Amanda, aged 24, drug user
No, I never used condoms with him 'cause, like, I had been with him for a bit and, like, we just never used them from the start, so I never did.

Angie, aged 22, non-drug user (sauna worker)
We have never used condoms. Once you get into this game, you don't use condoms outside. In the past, if I was to go out and meet somebody, say in a club, then yeah, it might have been condoms, but in this job, you don't really have one night stands, so because you are with people a bit longer, it means that you don't use condoms outside. I have had two relationships since I started doing this and I didn't use condoms with either of them. I don't think you go looking for one night stands when you are in this job, you have had enough of 'wham, bam, thank you mam' all bloody day and, let's face it, a one night stand is the same as a punter, only they are not paying for it!

In spite of these sentiments expressed by some women during the interviews, the data reveal that casual non-paying partners were a feature of the women's sexual activities: 82 per cent of drug users reported one or more other non-paying sexual partners in addition to their regular partner in the six months prior to interview, as did 74 per cent of non-drug users. Condom use with these partners was low for both groups of women, but non-users were significantly more likely to use condoms in these encounters (26 per cent as opposed to 9 per cent). An additional factor for drug users in these casual encounters was intoxication and memory loss. Many women described being too intoxicated to insist on condom use, or not even remembering much of what happened but feeling pretty sure that the man concerned would not have used a condom.

Data from the interviews with 120 male clients of female prostitutes provide some valuable insights into what sort of men use prostitutes on a regular basis and the risks they are prepared to take. The mean age of respondents to the study was 39 years old, ranging from 19 to 61 years. Twenty-nine per cent of the sample were single, 4 per cent separated, 8 per cent divorced and 3 per cent widowed. Fifty-six per cent of the sample were married and living with their wives. A further 12 men lived with their partner while not actually being married, bringing the total of those living with a regular female sexual partner to 62 per cent. However, 32 per cent of the sample did live entirely alone at the time of the interview and some members of this group clearly emphasised loneliness and an inability to make lasting sexual relationships as a reason for using prostitutes.

Unlike the female prostitutes, many of whom had never had what one might term a 'proper job', only 11 per cent of the male clients were unemployed, a figure in line with the overall rate of unemployment across the north west region. The most commonly described occupation was managerial (16 per cent), with 12 per cent describing their occupation as professional. The remainder of the sample had jobs mainly in white collar or skilled manual employment, while 12 per cent of respondents described themselves as self-employed.

The vast majority of men (67 per cent) reported contacting prostitutes in the street. In fact, many of those interviewed described having tried other ways of contacting prostitutes, i.e. saunas, and finding the 'thrill' was taken out of the encounter, even though their reputation was much more at risk on the streets. Those men who favoured contact magazines were all looking for specialist masochistic services: of those interviewed, the majority described having to find one or two women whom they could trust and who provided these services, as their sexual needs involved being tied up or put in other positions in which they would be open to exploitation. Twenty-two per cent of the sample reported favouring saunas as a means of contacting prostitutes, and a number of men interviewed mentioned the advantage of cleanliness, and knowing that the women were not drug users, as well as the minimal chance of being arrested, as the main reasons for this choice. Some of the men with very responsible managerial jobs were obviously using the saunas as a means of dealing with stress. One manager who was separated from his wife said that he could not talk to subordinates about problems but he could go to the saunas and tell the women anything and they would listen sympathetically.

Of the men who bought vaginal sex with prostitutes in the twelve months prior to interview, 62 per cent claimed to have always used a condom, 33 per cent said they sometimes did, and 5 per cent said never. For oral sex, the figures were: 40 per cent always, 50 per cent sometimes and 8 per cent never. For anal sex the figures were: 66 per cent always, 30 per cent sometimes and 4 per cent never. Condom use with regular sexual partners and wives was almost non-existent.

Interview data from the women's study also provided useful insights into who these men are and the attitudes of the women towards them.

Maria, aged 28, drug user

A lot of them are married. They come for things the wife won't do, or they come rather than have an affair – no commitment, you see . . . this is not going to lead to me wanting a wedding ring, is it? . . . I find they are mostly the business types, especially the ones who want domination stuff . . . I find they are the ones in the boss position. They dish it out all day, see, I think they like a bit back . . . It turns them on, a woman shouting at them.

Karine, aged 33, drug user

It's basically the young guy that is either on his way to a club or on his way home from a club. He can't be bothered with the chatting up. He doesn't want to pick up a girl, then all evening he pays for her drinks on the off chance she may or she may not; and if she does, the next time he's in that pub, she is giving him loads of hassle, like 'Why didn't you phone?' and all that. Or it's a married guy whose wife is pregnant or in the menopause or something, the middle-aged guy who is not sure he can still do it, you know.

Marta, aged 26, non-drug user

You get the one-offs as well who have never done it before, I mean never used a prostitute before; they are absolutely terrified and they have usually come before you have done anything because they have been driving round all night thinking about it, stupid sods. Well, you just have to think: Well, tough! You know what I mean? That's the attitude you have to have; I mean you are not going to give them a refund, are you?

Cathy, aged 21, drug user

You get the lads that will bring their mate down for his stag night and pay for him, you know. You get the really old man who will walk round for an hour talking to all the girls and then he will pick one. They are basically lonely, and he will pick the one who was the friendliest to him; she might have a face like the back of a bus, it won't matter, that will be the one he will go for.

Teresa, aged 27, drug user
In town, you get a lot of businessmen who are not particularly lonely; it's just that they want to try something other than the wife. They are away from home and it's all on expenses, paid for by the firm, she won't miss it from the housekeeping; you know the type.

Conclusions

The majority of female respondents had, over the previous year, been in contact with a number of health care agencies and professionals. Interestingly, however, the women reported a very low level of awareness in relation to their sexual activity on the part of professionals such as GPs, midwives and nurses working in genito-urinary medicine clinics.

Recent research studies examining attitudes of nurses to those with AIDS, such as those by Bond et al (1991) and Akinsanya and Rouse (1992), report a worrying inability on the part of nurses to discuss sex with their patients, especially where HIV is concerned. This stems not simply from lack of confidence: there are particular difficulties when the sexual orientation and the experience of the nurse differs from that of the patient. Nurses suffer from the confused sexual imagery which surrounds our profession, stretching from the asexual, motherly caring, nurturing image to the sexy nymph in suspenders and black stockings. A person's sexuality and the physical expression of it is an integral part of all relationships, yet nurses have been and still are expected to repress their own sexuality and to ignore that of their patients.

Everything connected with sexuality is burdened with what Lawler (1991) calls 'cultural baggage'. Most nurses are women and nursing activities often require a level of intimacy not usual outside sex. Sexual harassment of nurses is common and nursing has to deal with this in its everyday work and often does so in a maladaptive fashion. Isobel Menzies (1959) clearly described how this aspect of work causes many nurses, of course unconsciously, to split off aspects of the totality of the patient in order to be able to deal with the whole. Such 'destructive splitting' often leads to ill treatment, aggression and violence. Other people's sexuality challenges and disturbs our concepts of ourselves, and produces a great desire to place those people whose sexual behaviour or sexuality does not fit our 'norm' into some damaged or pathological category. Indeed, we need look no further than psychiatric textbooks from the not-so-distant past to find homosexuality under headings such as sexual deviance and psychopathy, along with prostitution and promiscuity.

If we find sex difficult to talk about as nurses, then 'risky sex' poses an even bigger problem. And it is this particular issue which highlights the danger to nursing in relation to HIV. There is an increasing lobby in the media and right-wing political circles who still refuse to see HIV as relevant to anyone who is not either gay, a drug user or a prostitute. Even for the so-called radical feminist wing, this problem with sex has led to claims that the 'AIDS crisis', with its attendant calls for a reduction in sexual activity outside of stable relationships, is a mere ploy to emphasise monogamy and force a return to 'family values'.

HIV requires that nursing wakes up fast to the need for sexuality awareness and stresses its importance in clinical supervision (Butterworth and Faugier 1993) in order to provide the best possible advice and care for our patients. Sexuality awareness is not, however, something reserved for others: all nurses, particularly those in positions of educational leadership, need to be honest and aware in respect of their own sexuality and the way it influences their ideas, teaching and research. Anything less would merely imply continued repression and a lack of integrity.

References

Akinsanya J A and Rouse P (1992) Who will care? A survey of the knowledge attitudes of hospital nurses to people with HIV/AIDS. *Journal of Advanced Nursing,* **17**, 400–401.

Araldsen T and Hansen B (1993) *Heterosexual women's vulnerability for HIV infection on intended and unintended consequences of sexuality.* 9th International Conference on AIDS, Berlin.

Bond S, Rhodes T, Phillips P, Setter J, Foy C and Bond J (1991) Experience and preparation of community nursing staff for work associated with HIV infection and AIDS. *Social Science and Medicine,* **32**, 1, 71–76.

Butterworth T, and Faugier J M (1993) *Clinical Supervision and Mentorship in Nursing.* London: Chapman & Hall.

Chin J (1990) Current and future dimensions of the HIV/AIDS pandemic in women and children. *Lancet,* **336**, 221–224.

Center for Disease Control (1992) *AIDS and antibody to human immunodeficiency virus infection in the United States. 1992 Update.* Atlanta: Center for Disease Control.

Darrow W W (1984) Prostitution and sexually transmitted disease. In Holmes K K, Mardh P A, Sparling P E and Weisner P J (eds) *Sexually transmitted diseases.* New York: McGraw Hill.

Day S and Ward H (1992) *Commercial sex and HIV risk: male partners of female sex workers.* 8th International Conference on AIDS, Amsterdam.

Doerr H W, Enzenberger R, Bolender C, Fischer S and Peters M (1990) *Prevalence of HIV infection in prostitutes from Frankfurt.* 6th International Conference on AIDS, San Francisco.

Elbaz G (1993) *Women do not get AIDS. They just die from it.* 9th International Conference on AIDS, Berlin.

Goffman E (1968) *Stigma – Notes on the Management of Spoiled Identity.* London: Pelican Books.

Goldberg D J, Green S T, Kingdom J C P and Christie P R (1988) HIV infection among female drug injecting prostitutes in Greater Glasgow. *Communicable Diseases Bulletin (Scotland),* **88**, 12, 1–3.

Hartgers C (1989) AIDS and drugs. *AIDS Care*, **1**, 206–211.

Holland J, Ramazanoglu C and Scott S et al (1990) Sex, gender and power: young women's sexuality in the shadow of AIDS. *Sociology of Health and Illness*, **12**, 3, 336–351.

Kinnel H (1989) *Prostitutes, their clients and risks of HIV infection in Birmingham*. Occasional Paper, Department of Public Health Medicine, Birmingham.

Klee H, Faugier J M, Hayes C, Boulton T and Morris J (1990) Factors associated with risk behaviour among injecting drug users. *AIDS Care*, **2**, 133–154.

Lawler J (1991) *Behind the Screens – Nursing and the Somology of the Body*. Edinburgh: Churchill Livingstone.

Marmor M, Des Jarlais D C, Cohen H et al (1987) Risk factors for infection with HIV among drug users in New York City. *AIDS*, **1**, 39–44.

McKeganey N and Barnard M (1992) *AIDS, Drugs and Sexual Risk – Lives in the Balance*. Milton Keynes: Open University Press.

Menzies I E P (1959) The functioning of social systems as a defence against anxiety: a report on a study of the nursing service of a general hospital. *Human Relations*, **13**, 95–121.

Morgan Thomas R (1990) AIDS risks, alcohol, drugs, and the sex industry: a Scottish study. In Plant M (ed.) *AIDS, Drugs and Prostitution*. London: Routledge.

Nichols E K (1989) *Mobilizing against AIDS*. Cambridge, Mass.: Harvard University Press.

Padian N S (1988) Prostitute women and AIDS: epidemiology. *AIDS*, **6**, 413–419.

Pateman C (1988) *The Sexual Contract*. Cambridge: Polity Press.

Plant M (1990) Sex work, alcohol, drugs and AIDS. In Plant M (ed.) *AIDS, Drugs and Prostitution*. London: Routledge.

Proceedings of the VIII International Conference on AIDS and the III STD World Congress. Amsterdam, The Netherlands, 19–24 July 1992.

Richardson D (1989) *Women and the AIDS crisis*. London: Pandora.

Robertson R (1987) *Heroin, AIDS and Society*. London: Hodder and Stoughton.

Scrambler G, Peswani R, Renton A et al (1990) Women prostitutes in the AIDS era. *Sociology of Health and Illness*, **12**, 3, 260–274.

Sontag S (1991) *Illness as Metaphor. AIDS and its Metaphors*. Harmondsworth: Penguin Books.

Tirrelli U, Rezza G, Guillani M (1989) HIV seroprevalence among 304 female prostitutes from four Italian towns. *AIDS*, **3**, 547–548.

Verrisimo J, Pucheu D and Morais C A (1993) *Bio-psychosocial profile of women who contracted HIV through sexual intercourse with steady partners*. 9th International Conference on AIDS, Berlin.

Ward H, Day S, Donegan C and Harris J R W (1990) *HIV risk behaviour and STD incidence in London prostitutes*. 6th International conference on AIDS, San Francisco.

Weeks J (1989) AIDS: the intellectual agenda. In Aggleton P, Hart G and Davies P (eds), *AIDS: Social Representations, Social Practices*. Lewis: Falmer Press.

World Health Organization (1992) *Global AIDS statistics: 31st Dec 92*. Geneva: World Health Organization.

Chapter 5
Community Care for People Living with HIV/AIDS
Pat Turton

For the homosexual community AIDS has been a holocaust. The spiteful laws and mean prejudice which supports homophobia enable our society to deny the inherent, and essential, sexuality of all human beings. A society which collectively still views sexuality as an embarrassing personality flaw is not well placed to protect itself from AIDS (Paul, a patient's partner).

Introduction

This chapter draws on a study I conducted as a practitioner/researcher in the period 1989–91. From my background in anthropology and district nursing I was concerned to establish what changes, if any, in service provision would enable people with HIV-related illness to be cared for at home, if that was their choice, and to bring about or facilitate such changes. Gay men represented the overwhelming majority of HIV positive patients in the research locality. In this chapter, therefore, I focus on gay men with HIV disease and discuss issues and concerns related to sexuality as they affected the provision of primary health care; lay carers (families, partners and friends); and the patient – physically, mentally and socially throughout the illness.

Although not limited to the male homosexual community, the HIV virus has affected this community in the UK disproportionately. HIV/AIDS was, therefore, linked from the start with 'sexuality', or more precisely, homosexuality. AIDS was dubbed by the tabloid press 'the gay plague'. 'AIDS is understood in a premodern way . . . which also revives the archaic idea of a tainted community that illness had judged' (Sontag 1988). In both Britain and America, homosexuals remain the largest category of people affected by the virus to date. It is the various psychological and social aspects associated with sexuality and this client group, as much as the disease itself, which make it different from other illnesses and which particularly affect its management in

the community (George 1988, Catalan 1989, Schofferman 1989). Problems
with home care arise largely from the unavoidable fact that, as Carney puts it,

> Once you take AIDS care out of an institutional setting and move it into
> the community, you must add that community's dynamics to the picture.
>
> (Carney 1990, 33)

AIDS and Community Care

The association between AIDS and homophobia has been responsible, to
some extent, for the slow acceptance of the principle that people with HIV/
AIDS could and should be cared for in the community (King 1987).
GPs lacked confidence in their knowledge of HIV (Lande 1988, Kilbane,
O'Donnell and McKnight 1989). More importantly, GPs may have negative
attitudes towards people with AIDS, especially homosexuals (Boyton and
Scrambler 1988, Milne and Keene 1988, Sibbald and Freeling 1988). A study
from North East Thames and Berkshire, for example, found that one in six
GPs in the sample thought that AIDS could only be controlled by recriminalis-
ing homosexuality and 10 per cent 'would not disagree with the statement that
homosexuality should be made illegal' (Singh 1991). It is, therefore, hardly
surprising that, as King notes

> Fear of stigmatisation has prevented people at risk for AIDS from fully
> explaining their sexual behaviour and lifestyle to doctors. Patients perceive
> accurately or inaccurately, their GPs as having particular attitudes to sexual
> orientation and this will affect the degree of self disclosure that they are
> prepared to make.
>
> (King 1987, 1)

People with HIV avoid contact with community services as a consequence
of this perceived homophobia combined with lack of confidence in GPs'
knowledge about the disease (King 1987). In a cohort study of homosexual
patients Roderick and Stevens (1989) found that patients had difficulties in
dealing with their own GPs and utilised the acute hospitals for all their care.
In a study of London patients Mansfield and Singh (1989) reported that over
half the sample were either not registered with a GP or were unwilling to
disclose information to the GP, especially regarding AIDS-related symptoms.
   A substantial minority of community nursing staff, like their GP colleagues,
have negative feelings towards caring for people who are HIV positive, and
particularly those whose behaviour puts them at risk of HIV infection (Bond
et al 1988). Indeed, sexuality has been identified by the Ministerial AIDS
Action group as an issue which causes problems for a range of health care
professionals. Two aspects, they found, were of particular concern to the
individual worker – first, their inability 'to acknowledge, or feel comfortable
with, the topic of sexuality when faced with clients/patients', and secondly,

'the inadequacies in professional education and training relating to sexuality' (ENB 1993). Smith's study (1989) confirms the link between UK nurses' attitudes to homosexuality and their willingness to care for a gay patient. Ninety-seven per cent of her random sample of 50 district nurses viewed haemophiliacs as 'not deserving to get AIDS'. A quarter of the sample, however, considered that homosexuals 'deserve' to get AIDS and over half suggested that their 'immoral behaviour' had caused the illness (Smith 1989). It has been argued that prejudice among nurses towards 'high risk groups' perpetuates an unreasonable fear of contagion and leads to 'a shunning of those afflicted' (Gallagher 1990). Such negative attitudes towards homosexuals are arguably a constraint to providing effective HIV care by UK community nurses, for as Bond et al, commenting on the findings of their national study on community nurses and HIV, note:

> Whilst the proportion of staff who were of the opinion that they should have the right to refuse to deal with certain patients were in the minority, they may still give rise to concern. Patients' perceptions of nursing staff may depend upon the effects created by negative opinions of such a minority of nursing staff rather than the positive, but often less newsworthy, opinions of the majority. In this event the relationship potential between nurses and patients may suffer.
>
> (Bond et al 1988, 131)

The association between sexuality and AIDS has, on the other hand, created an active civil rights-style response to which many nurses have rallied. Such nurses become involved not only in direct patient care services provided by the voluntary associations but also in prevention, education and political activities (Mostert 1991). Indeed, 'from the earliest days of the epidemic, nurses have assumed strong roles in developing such volunteer and community based AIDS services, and as care providers within them' (Fox, Aiken and Messikomer 1990). Nurses have, for example, 'been pivotally involved in the Gay Men's Health Crisis' (Fox et al 1990) since it was founded in New York in 1982. And it was they who have been particularly notable in

> detailing gaps and shortfalls in service provision, monitoring and attempting to correct how persons with AIDS were being treated by health care professionals, and providing advice through a hotline and a variety of counselling and direct care services.
>
> (Kobasa 1990, 283)

Gay men are generally able to rely on the support of friends in time of need and illness (Brendstrup and Schmidt 1990, Hart and Fitzpatrick 1990, Raveis and Seigel 1991, McCann and Wadsworth 1992, Britton, Zarski and Hobfall 1993). For many AIDS patients, however, as George and Hart note 'the assumption that there is a base line of primary care which will come from the "family" is not realistic' (George and Hart 1989). Support by gay partners and friends forms a fragile care unit that cannot, therefore, be relied on over time. For, as Raveis notes, 'as the epidemic progresses and friendship groups become attenuated by the disease, this source of social support is likely to diminish' (Raveis and Seigel 1991, 41).

Unfortunately, however, Morgan notes 'that the social network of gay partners may actually dry up because the emotional and concrete demands are too threatening, too time consuming, or too unsolvable for friends to handle' (Morgan and Rogers 1993, 11). Isolation, loneliness and often the additional burden of having to conceal their care-giving and grief from employers and the wider community leave lovers very vulnerable to stress (Raveis and Seigel 1991, Morgan and Rogers 1993). Indeed, Lynch (1977) has documented how 'loneliness and isolation can literally "break your heart"'.

Desire for support and 'closeness' may be taken to an extreme extent and result in HIV negative partners of patients actively and intentionally infecting themselves from their lovers in what has been described as a modern day version of the Romeo and Juliet suicide pact (Morgan and Rogers 1993). Even if such an extreme response is rejected by an HIV negative partner, the diagnosis will have a considerable impact on the dynamics of their sexual relationship. An HIV diagnosis, as Flaskerud notes,

> requires a change in sexual activities both to avoid transmission and infection and in response to decreased sexual desires because of illness. All of these changes in relationship can be intensely stressful and demoralising to the spouse/lover.
>
> (Flaskerud 1989, 159)

The need for financial and physical support may be the impetus for the gay HIV positive man to reconnect with his family or origin (Britton and Zarski 1989) and overcome any rift his sexual orientation may have caused in their relationship (Stables 1990). When a gay man in late-stage HIV disease recontacts his biological family the members are 'suddenly confronted with enormous demands'. These care-givers, primarily parents and siblings, are as Raveis and Seigel suggest, 'frequently unprepared for such challenges and require emotional support in dealing with the illness' (Raveis and Seigel 1991, 41).

Family support for gay men is, therefore, complicated by sexuality issues; an issue that, in this context, concerns gay patients' partners is the definition of 'family' and 'next of kin' (Librach 1988, Bor 1990, Wilkie 1992). This is particularly problematic if the patient is confused or unconscious and has not made a will or given clear instruction as to whom he wishes to be recognised as next of kin (Librach 1988). Even if the partner has been nominated as the next of kin and is therefore recognised as such by the hospital, the patient's family may find this difficult to accept (King 1989).

Illness and Treatment Effects

The Asymptomatic Phase

When first tested HIV positive, usually in the asymptomatic phase, the gay patient's psychosocial reactions to diagnosis are 'similar to those seen in other potentially fatal conditions, but they are magnified by the stigma attached and by fears of social rejection' (Catalan 1989). Patients may internalise the predominant culture's homophobia and feel negatively about their own sexuality. Depression is frequently associated with self blame (Miller 1986). Even people, as Anderson points out,

> who do not ordinarily have problems concerning their sexual identity might well have temporary problems that result from the stress of receiving an HIV anti-body positive diagnosis, or a diagnosis of HIV related illness, which adds a new stigma to face and overcome . . . and may feel some guilt about their sexuality.
>
> (Anderson 1992, 206)

The Early Symptomatic Phase

The consequences of an HIV diagnosis for the sexuality of gay men can be discussed under two headings: (a) conceptual disturbance and (b) functional disturbance (Miller 1986). Conceptual disturbance can include a very wide range of problems given that for many gay men, as Miller (1986) maintains, 'sexual activity is of central importance . . . as a means of homosexual affirmation'. With abstinence from 'easy' sexual activity, the patient may suffer a loss of his sexual identity, group affirmation and the social life connected with gay bars and clubs. The need to practise safe sex may, therefore, have indirect and often seriously debilitating consequences for the patient's own sexuality. Functional disturbance includes an initial loss of libido and/or erectile dysfunction, together with behaviour difficulties following from suggested guidelines for safer sex. Physical problems directly related to sexuality occur increasingly with the progress of the disease. Sexual dysfunction in HIV positive gay men has been associated with immune function, endocrine, neurological and psychiatric factors. Decreased sexual desire has been found to be significantly correlated to decreased T4 helper cell count, while impaired erectile and orgasmic function may be related to neurological conditions, especially peripheral neuropathy and psychiatric symptoms (Meyer-Bahlburg 1993). In a Canadian study (Cohen, Salit and Emott 1993) a mildly symptomatic group and those with AIDS reported high frequencies of an erectile disorder (40 per cent and 12.5 per cent) and hypoactive sexual desire disorder (40 per cent and 25 per cent). Cohen et al conclude that 'sexual dysfunctions increase significantly in gay men with symptomatic HIV illness' and that 'as quality of life issues are important . . . identifying and treating those with sexual dysfunction is worthwhile'.

Late Stage HIV Disease and Terminal Care

With the progress of the disease the patient experiences numerous debilitating and often disfiguring conditions which affect sexual function. For example, minor skin disorders, experienced by the majority of HIV positive people, may have a significant negative effect on self-esteem and sexual life. Sometimes these are exacerbations of previous skin disease but more often they are new to the patient. A papulopruritic eruption or 'itchy folliculitis', affecting much of the body surface, is one of the commonest skin problems in HIV disease and Farthing, Brown and Staughton (1988) note 'they are intensely pruritic and very frequently excoriated'. Seborrhoeic dermatitis is also very common.

Summarising the affects of three common, clinically serious HIV related syndromes Raveis and Seigel note that:

> Patients with Kaposi's sarcoma and their care givers live with a constant visual reminder of the disease. In the AIDS wasting syndrome, the dramatic weight loss markedly changes physical appearance and functioning. In the later stages of the disease course, patients may develop AIDS dementia complex, characterised by cognitive, motor, and behaviour dysfunctions.
>
> (Raveis and Seigel 1991, 41)

An undesirable change in body image, whether due to surgical intervention or some other alteration in physical appearance, is known to impact negatively on an individual's sexuality and self esteem (Webb 1985). For any patient with HIV disease the ability to maintain a positive body image is under constant threat. For a gay patient, body image changes may be a particularly upsetting phenomenon. Indeed Hay maintains that:

> in the gay culture extreme worship of youth and beauty add to the difficulties . . . If one is beautiful when he is young, he is adored and fussed over. Those not so attractive are made to feel as outsiders and never quite acceptable.
>
> (Hay 1988, 176)

The Study

Data for my study were generated by participant observation and informal tape-recorded interviews. Fieldwork was carried out over a two-year period while I was working as a practitioner/researcher. The study population included 55 gay late-stage HIV disease patients and their carers. Over the two-year study period, I formed close relationships with the people involved in the study. Situations and incidents, often concerning issues of sexuality, were recorded in fieldnotes. Often distressing, these incidents were later reviewed and their significance discussed with the patient and/or carer, when possible during tape-recorded informal interviews. In some instances patients or carers wrote their own accounts of their experience for the study.

Themes related to sexuality that emerged from the study can be subsumed under the three headings used to discuss the literature. They relate, therefore, to the impact of concerns related to sexuality on, first, the provision of primary health care; second, lay carers – families, partners and friends; and, last but not least, the patient – physically, mentally and socially throughout the course of his illness.

Provision of Primary Health Care

Patients, at the start of my fieldwork period in late 1989, voiced the opinion that utilising GP services was neither necessary nor desirable. As one patient, Adam, put it 'I don't feel you have to have a GP . . : a lot of people I know don't have GPs. If they have any problems they go straight to where they are being treated and get sorted out there'. The perceived homophobic attitudes of GPs were a key element in this decision. Adam, for example, explained that he had

> heard horror stories about GPs and how they have treated people. There is a lot of prejudice there. I know things have changed now and there is a lot of education in the system and people have become more aware of the issues about HIV, but, having said that, there are still GPs who are the same as before.

Fifteen of the 55 gay patients in my study had no GP when initially contacted. A survey of 122 patients (Ong et al 1993) undertaken in the same locality during 1989, found that only 20 (16 per cent) indicated that their GP was aware of their HIV status. An overwhelming majority, 84 per cent of the sample, did not want their GP involved in their care. Lack of confidentiality (66 per cent) and lack of expertise (34 per cent) were given as the reasons for this decision. King, however, in a study of out patients attending HIV clinics in London, found that one of the principal reasons for withholding information about their HIV status was 'a fear of a negative reaction from the doctor' (King 1989, 140). In my study, patients (whose GP was aware of their status) focused less on 'confidentiality' and 'expertise' as reasons for not involving GPs in their care, than on the reality (validating the anticipatory fear expressed by King's sample) of the negative response they had received when their doctor first learnt of their diagnosis. Describing his experience Adam, who was tested without his knowledge or consent, said:

> I received a letter from my GP telling me that I was HIV positive. I just couldn't believe it. I thought it was automatically AIDS and that I would die. I was just blown – distraught. And when I went to see my GP he was off hand. He did not want to see me. He was busy. Said there was nothing he could do. Perhaps I had got two years at the most.

Such lack of compassion was perceived by patients as evidence of anti-gay feeling and a sufficient reason to avoid involving the GP. As a consequence of this, Adam noted that 'a lot of people want to die at home, but they don't want community nursing services'. This refusal was not related to the acceptability of the nurse but rather an avoidance of involvement with the GP. Patients, he maintained, 'have an idea that community nurses have to report back to the GP. There is a breach of confidentiality – the GP would find out. So that puts a stop on a lot of people'.

Patients recognised that GPs lacked an understanding of gay sexuality and partnership as approximating marriage. GPs were felt, therefore, to be unable to support gay men appropriately. Darryl and his partner Ben, for example, went into the GPs room to hear Ben's test result. The doctor asked Darryl to leave the room. Darryl reflected:

> I left but now I wish I hadn't. It was a problem we both had to face as a couple. But the doctor did not really understand our feelings for each other . . . The doctor was totally inexperienced to deal with the situation he was in. He was upset and embarrassed. He could offer no support.

Given time, however, some GPs proved to be a major support to their HIV patients. As another partner, Paul, put it about his initially 'reluctant GP', he became able 'to talk with the same level of camaraderie as one would imagine he would use when talking to a close friend at the golf club'. Likewise Darryl, reflecting on the night Ben died, recalled how:

> the GP came as soon as possible. He gave him morphine to kill the pain. By this time Ben had soiled the bed. It was an absolute mess. Me and our doctor cleaned him and changed his bed. It was a long night but the GP was wonderful.

In contrast to GPs, patients did not anticipate that district nurses would hold negative attitudes towards gay men. They were, however, concerned that they would be stigmatised on account of their diagnosis. 'We were', said Darryl, 'so afraid of how people would react, even professional people such as nurses, to our medical condition'. Months later, having eventually agreed to use the district nurses, he noted, with evident relief, that:

> They were marvellous, kind, caring and helpful. They couldn't have given a damn what Ben was dying of, he was just another patient who needed care. Why didn't we use them sooner? I wish we had, but we were frightened.

Reasons for refusing community nursing care were related almost entirely to the fear that such involvement would lead to breaches in confidentiality, either to the GP or to the wider community. Patients were concerned about the effect of such breaches not only on themselves but, as significantly, on their partners. In some cases this had dire consequences. Relating the story of a close friend, Adam said:

He had KS. It was all over him. I had even gone into his foot and his foot was breaking open. The pain he was going through must have been terrible but he would not have community services. He lived with his partner and he was thinking of his partner afterwards – having to put up with all the stick. People who are terminally ill think, at the end of the day, it's finished for them. But it's the beginning for their partner. They tend to protect their partners and this is a way of protecting them – by not having community nurses.

Harassment for being gay was a common and frequent experience of patients. Uniformed district nurses visiting the home would, it was believed, exacerbate the problem by, as Adam put it:

creating a breach of confidentiality. Not by them but by what people think. People put two and two together. When you walk down the street they say, 'there's them two queers'. Because we're 'queer' if a nurse came to see us they'd assume one of us has AIDS. So we just can't have community nursing.

Lay Carers – Families, Partners and Friends

Fear of infection, concern over the patient's homosexuality, grieving and sheer physical exhaustion affect lay carers' sexuality. For gay partners the stress is particularly great. Many know themselves to be HIV positive and a significant minority of them are symptomatic. Others choose not to be tested and live instead with their anxiety and the knowledge that 'it is impossible to retrospectively reduce the risk'. One such partner, Paul, describing the particular configuration of fear, exhaustion and isolation that partners of patients experience, said:

Only through the support of my partner, Vincent, was I able to avoid going completely crazy. The impact of living almost permanently in a state of high anxiety was considerable. Once he had been diagnosed my anxiety about AIDS was substantially replaced by the anxiety about him and the over-riding need to give him support, help and care. Although I could not share the physical pain I could on another level share the emotional experience. Over the last three years I have provided almost 24 hours a day care. This is an incredibly taxing and lonely way to spend one's life.

Paul was supported in his grief by both his own and his partner's family, but none the less he felt very lonely and isolated without Vincent. A year after Vincent's death Paul was found dead in their double bed. He was 40 years old. Cause of death was recorded as 'cardiac ischaemia'. His family believe that he died of a broken heart.

In many cases, however, family support for bereaved partners was not forthcoming. Frequently kin, aware of the relationship between their son/ brother and his lover, neither acknowledged nor accepted it. This situation was often compounded by the manner in which the patient had dealt over time with his sexuality and partnership in relation to his family. Mark's way, for example, was to create a smoke-screen for his family to avoid any possibility that they would find out about his sexual preferences or HIV status. When Mark died, his partner Toby explained:

> He always kept his gayness away from his family. He was ashamed of it. He kept contact with his family. But I was never allowed to go and see them, although I said I wanted to meet them. He didn't feel the family could cope with it or the fact that he had HIV. He always had some reason why he was poorly . . . it was flu or something . . . So we detached ourself from the family, both mine and his. He wanted to keep it secret – so I had to keep it secret. It was a combination of both being gay and having AIDS.

Additional stress is caused by the legal difficulties surrounding gay partners' inheritance rights and 'next of kin' status. Toby, for example, was in a situation where his lover's family disapproved of homosexuality. When they found out about Mark and Toby's relationship they were 'disgusted' and disparaging of the love between the pair: 'we would have felt differently if you were a woman but you are not!'. They threatened to challenge Toby's right to be 'next of kin' in a court of law. Toby explained, once the situation had been amicably resolved, that

> It was important to be next of kin. Because I did feel married to Mark. We were together for 7 years and always with each other except during work. I would like to see gay marriages if it was to save the wrangle at the end. Something a bit more legal has to be sorted out.

Apart from gay partners, the majority of carers were the patients' parents. Mothers represented the overwhelming majority of carers besides gay partners and their feelings were similar to those of mothers who had lost their sons in battle. O'Casey (1980) encapsulates the essence of their grief with the words 'What was the pain I suffered, Johnny, bringing you into the world to carry you to your cradle, to the pain I'll suffer carryin' you out of the world to bring you to your grave'.

Patients – Physically, Mentally and Socially

HIV-related wasting creates premature ageing and a cachectic appearance; the plaques of Kaposi's sarcoma (KS) can obliterate the features, and other skin conditions, such as severe molluscum contagiosum, are cosmetically difficult to conceal. Such visible signs of HIV have a major effect not only on the patient's self-image but on his sexual and social relations. Extreme weight loss was perceived by Simon, for example, as the cause of his boyfriend's rejection and his own loss of libido. He said:

> I've lost a hell of a lot of weight. I'm 6 foot 2 inches. I'm 8 stone now and I was 14 stone. It stops me buying clothes and the sex goes. I can do with being cuddled, but no sex. My boyfriend told me my body made him feel sick. I was so skinny. That's why he didn't touch me. I felt really hurt. He even told my mother. He told her we were finished. When she asked him why, he said, 'well could you touch that body?'

To combat the problem of weight loss patients may be prescribed Megastrol, a progestational agent which is reported to suppress endogenous testosterone (Jekot and Purdy 1993). This can adversely affect the patient's sexuality by causing erectile dysfunction. Most patients were aware that 'it's female hormone'. As one 47-year-old said:

> It's bound to affect you. I've grown 'boobs'. I find achieving an erection is hard, no pun intended, achieving orgasm is harder – but it can be done. Anyway that's not as important in a sense to me. I'm older – I'm not chasing sex. I still have sex – but it's less of a drive.

His younger friend had 'stopped taking them because although it put on the weight, it mucked up his sex life. So he stopped taking it because his sex life is more important than putting on weight'.

Treatment that requires a permanent venous access, by inserting a cannula such as a Hickman line, creates an additional threat to the patient's body image. Voicing the feelings of many patients when describing his situation and its effect on his sense of sexuality, Vincent said:

> I have a problem with what is called in the jargon 'body image'. I have always had an attractive body. I enjoy the physicality and inherent sensuality of feeling and looking attractive. (Even the ravages of AIDS have not yet obliterated this.) A Hickman line may not look bad, particularly to medical professionals, but I was the person who was going to have to live with it. And in my perception it would make me an adjunct to a plastic tube. Age and AIDS reduces one's physical attractiveness (both with alarming rapidity) but a Hickman line can be a very abrupt transition.

Vincent's concern with 'body image' was such that he was prepared to go blind in preference to having a long line inserted in order to have the necessary i.v. therapy for his cytomegalovirus (CMV) retinitis. Vincent's choice was not, he maintained, 'motivated by fear. It was not bloody minded. It was an exercise of my free will'.

Apart from the effects of the illness itself, and the associated treatment, the behavioural changes expected of the HIV positive patient affect his sexual relations. For some patients, becoming HIV positive leads to feelings of guilt about their sexual orientation and a consequent loss of libido. For many, however, sexual expression remained a vital force in their lives. As Howard put it:

> I try to be positive about living with AIDS. I don't let it spoil my enjoyment of life – and sex. I'm not promiscuous and I only have relations with HIV positive men. I'd like a monogamous relationship – so I'm answering ads in the personal column of the BP magazine.

In what is known as 'a magnetic couple', that is where one of the partners is HIV positive and the other negative, the need to practise safe sex is a crucial concern. Responsibility for this is usually a burden placed on the positive partner, often in the face of the negative partner's opposition. Describing his own position Adam said:

> It's difficult at times, but it's down to me as an individual. I still have a fear of infecting him but he feels differently. He feels that our relationship should be the same as it was. He says he's not really bothered about becoming infected. All I keep thinking about is if he were to become infected I wouldn't be able to forgive myself. Even though it would be his choice as well. It would be something I would have to carry and I don't think I would carry it very well. I have told him we are going to carry on having 'safer sex', it's as simple as that. But it sometimes causes a bit of trauma. It's very hard. Sometimes you feel you're going towards an unsafe act and you have to snap out of it quick. Get behind me Satan! Yes it's very difficult sometimes.

Despite good intentions Adam's partner was tested HIV positive eighteen months later.

Sexuality Related Nursing Care for HIV Patients

Carers, partners, parents and friends play a central role in enabling HIV patients to remain at home. District nurses are likely to be among the few people that patients and their lay carers trust and can share their anxiety with. District nurses, then, are in a prime position to identify and alleviate concerns and problems and, as my study has shown, these may include:

Psychological problems
 Anticipatory grief, sadness, loss, body image concerns
 Anxiety – panic attacks, insomnia
 Anger at injustice/guilt (AIDS = Anger Inappropriately Directed at Self)
 Depression, disturbance of mood, suicide

Physical problems
  Susceptibility to infection
  Nausea, vomiting, diarrhoea and constipation
  Respiratory distress
  Weakness and fatigue
  Skin problems/breakdown
  Pain
  Confusion, dementia
  Paralysis
  Blindness

Social problems
  Stigma
  Loneliness
  Family conflict
  Work and insurance
  Financial problems
  Housing

Nursing Interventions

Many sexuality-related problems, at every stage of the disease, are amenable to nursing interventions and can be considered as primary, secondary and tertiary health promotion.

Primary health promotion to maintain well-being
Neither general nor specific sexuality-related health promotion will be successful unless the patient can realistically cooperate with advice, for example, about diet. It is essential, therefore, for nurses to promote the health of the HIV positive person by ensuring that they are in receipt of the cash benefits to which they are entitled and that they have adequate heat and housing.

Secondary health promotion to reduce the risk of new infections
Lang summarises the measures that should be taken to maximise well-being and reduce the risk of new infection in the HIV positive patient. They include explaining the need for 'safe sex' even between positive partners to 'protect against possible re-infection with a more virulent form of HIV and against other sexually transmitted diseases' (Lang 1993). Stopping smoking, moderation of alcohol consumption and general physical fitness programmes should be supported by nurses. Scrupulous food, dental and personal hygiene should be emphasised to reduce the immune compromised person's exposure to

potentially harmful bacteria. A high-calorie, high-protein diet should be encouraged to combat actual or potential weight loss and maximise resistance to infection. Commonly, people with HIV are committed to maintaining their health and weight at optimum levels as a positive act of self-help and seek encouragement in this from nurses.

Encouraging patients to join an AIDS voluntary association is often beneficial. Such organisations offer 'an opportunity for empowerment, an orientation toward self and world that allows one effectively to respond to the many stressors of contemporary life' (Kobasa 1990).

Tertiary health promotion to minimise the effects of illness when they occur
The availability of effective treatments for a number of opportunistic infections has, as noted earlier, improved both the quality of life and life expectancy for HIV positive patients. Following an acute infection patients will, however, often have residual disability and/or require life-long prophylactic treatment. Community nurses can play a major role in dealing with symptoms that are of particular concern for patients' sexuality and affect their quality of life, for example, improving sleeping patterns, enhancing appetite and maintaining their nutritional status.

Unintended weight loss is one of the classic symptoms associated with AIDS patients, indeed 'chronic wasting syndrome', in which an HIV positive patient loses 10 or more per cent of his body weight, plus either diarrhoea or fever for one month is diagnostic of AIDS. Patients who are depressed or anxious may lack appetite and need encouragement to eat a well-balanced, high calorie diet (Peck and Johnson 1990). Even 'well-adjusted' patients found that 'AIDS and medications manage to reduce even a robust appetite to nil'. Loss of appetite may be due to a number of contributing factors, such as alterations in taste, nausea or difficulty in swallowing as a result of oesophagitis. It may be due to a sore mouth caused by aphthous ulceration, gingivitis or oral Kaposi's sarcoma – often exacerbated by the effects of radiotherapy. The most common condition affecting the mouth, however, is *Candida albicans*. Nutrition supplements are usually recommended to people with a 10 per cent decrease in their weight. Having access to a liquidizer, a freezer and a microwave facilitates food preparation and processing and such equipment can usually be obtained from AIDS charities.

Skin problems are among the most distressing of HIV-related conditions. These include molluscum contagiosum and fungal infections of the skin and nails such as tinea. Seborrhoeic dermatitis is common and severe in HIV, often covering most of the person's face. Itchy folliculitis (papulopruritic eruption) can 'drive a person crazy'. Likewise dry skin (xeroderma) which is almost universal in AIDS patients is associated with intense itching. The regular use of moisturising creams (e.g. E45 and bath oils) can often give people considerable relief, at least from the itching.

Pain is also a frequently experienced symptom (Sims and Moss 1991) and in some cases it is compounded by the medication. Zidovudine (AZT) and ganciclovir (DHPG) may cause myalgia (muscle pain) and many of the drugs can cause headaches, nausea and gastrointestinal disturbance. Pain can cause major changes in patients' self-concept and ability to cope and therefore adversely affects patients' sexuality. Complementary/alternative therapy is very acceptable to people with HIV. In a national study Robinson and Maynard (1991) found that one in five of their sample of HIV positive people had used an alternative therapy such as massage, meditation, relaxation and aromatherapy and 46 per cent had made purchases from herbalists and health food shops. The proliferation of alternative therapies offered as treatments for AIDS (Chaitow and Martin 1988) and the lack of scepticism on the part of some patients, however, poses problems for community nurses who have to:

> walk a fine line between support for the patient and encouraging him or her to choose foolish and expensive alternative treatments just to foster the patient's sense of autonomy.
>
> (White 1989, 12).

Fear and anxiety accompany every new symptom with devastating damage to individuals' sense of control and sexuality. Having AIDS has been described as 'being awake in your own worst nightmare'. Being able to support hope in the face of AIDS by 'reminding individuals of the strengths that they possess to cope with difficulties' (Anderson 1992) is the prime contribution of the nurse to maintaining patients' and carers' self-esteem and sexuality. Creating a positive approach in a situation of uncertainty and loss is aided by the nurse 'just being there'. In a situation seen as hopeless, patients 'may sink into a depressive despair, whereby they become unable to mount appropriate psychological and physical defences against the illness' (King 1987). Lack of hope, it is argued, accelerates the patient's decline (Jourard 1970). Conversely, the health promotion role of nurses is to support patients in looking optimistically and realistically to the future. Nurses can sustain hope and 'hope allows the individual to use a crisis as an opportunity for growth' (Miller 1985). Providing accurate information, a non-judgmental approach, grief counselling and an introduction to a peer support group are the most valued interventions the nurse can offer people with HIV and their carers (Hannon 1990).

Sexuality is an essential part of 'hope' and personal growth, the preservation and enhancement of which is the ultimate goal of nursing care in the community. Community nurses can nurture individual patients' and carers' 'transition from being weak and vulnerable – to functioning – to living as fully as possible, (Miller 1985, 23). Humour is an essential element in this process. As Paul said 'Love of life, sense of humour and common sense have made an immeasurable contribution to my quality of life . . . if you could not laugh at it you could not carry on'.

Supporting Carers

Gay male carers who are HIV positive themselves merit particular attention. Awareness of their health needs and the toll that the physical and psychological burden of caring entails is vital. Validating positive partners' sexuality and the love they demonstrate towards their partner can make their burden easier to bear. Above all, community nurses help to maintain carers' sexuality by encouraging and facilitating their continuing enjoyment of life despite HIV, in whichever way possible. Use of 'gallows humour', by both patients and carers, for example, 'I've got a season ticket to the crem,' or 'don't I look great for a dying man' and 'don't bother to talk to him – he's past his sell by date' may require some 'getting used to' by the nurse.

Supporting carers through the process of death and grieving is quintessentially the community nurses' role in HIV care. Differences in this process from, for example, that associated with a death from cancer, result primarily from the stigma of AIDS. In addition the youth of the patient and the difficulties associated with his sexual orientation create a unique configuration of problems and stresses in carers. Nurses' support and counselling are vital in encouraging the bereaved to, in Worden's words, 'make a healthy withdrawal from the deceased and to feel comfortable reinvesting that emotion in another relationship' (Worden 1983). Awareness of 'abnormal grief reactions' and 'complicated mourning' of gay bereaved partners will alert nurses to problems. In some cases nurses will need to refer the patient to a specialist for assistance.

HIV negative partners are particularly vulnerable. They may suffer 'survivor guilt', a 'strong sense of isolation' and 'suicidal ideation' (Morgan and Rogers 1993). It is, therefore, critical for nurses to assess partners for risk of suicide and, as Morgan suggests, 'directly confront the HIV negative partner regarding self destructive behaviour if we are to prevent additional loss of life to AIDS' (Morgan and Rogers 1993). Affirming the love and care the partner gave to the deceased and acknowledging the normality of the partner's desire, and ability, to form new loving relationships in the future facilitates a positive adaptation to the loss. The bereaved partner who isolates himself from the gay community may forfeit not only opportunities to express his sexuality but, perhaps more significantly, a major source of support. While remembering dead lovers, for the surviving partner (HIV positive or negative) 'life must go on' and expressing sexuality is part of life.

References

Anderson C (1992) Gay men and HIV. *Reflective Helping in HIV and AIDS*, 198–214. Milton Keynes: Open University Press.
Bond S, Rhodes T, Philips P, Setters J, Foy C and Bond J (1988) A national study of HIV infection/AIDS and community nursing staff in England. University of Newcastle upon Tyne Health Care Research Unit.
Bor R (1990) The family and HIV/AIDS. *AIDS Care*, 2, 4, 409–412.
Boyton R and Scambler C (1988) Survey of general practitioners' attitudes to AIDS in the North West Thames and East Anglian Regions. *British Medical Journal*, 296, 538–540.
Brendstrup E and Schmidt K (1990) Homosexual and bisexual men coping with the AIDS epidemic. *Social Science and Medicine*, 30, 6, 713–720.

Britton P J and Zarski J J (1989) HIV spectrum disorders and the family. *AIDS Care*, **1**, 1, 85–92.

Britton P J, Zarski J J and Hobfall S E (1993) Psychological distress and the role of significant others in a population of gay/bisexual men in the era of HIV. *AIDS Care*, **5**, 1, 43–54.

Carney K L (1990) AIDS care comes home: balancing benefits and difficulties. *Home Healthcare Nurse*, **8**, 2, 32–37.

Catalan J (1989) HIV disease and psychiatric practice. *Psychiatric Bulletin*, **13**, 316–332.

Chaitow L and Martin S (1988) *A World Without AIDS: The Controversial Holistic Health Plan*. Wellingborough: Thorsons Publishing Group.

Cohen M, Salit I E and Emott S (1993) *Sexual dysfunctions in HIV-positive gay men*. IXth International Conference on AIDS, Berlin.

ENB (1993) Sexual health education: breaking down the barriers. *AIDSet* 7, 1.

Farthing C, Brown S and Staughton R (1988) *A Colour Atlas of AIDS and HIV Disease*. Ipswich: Wolfe Medical Publications Ltd.

Flaskerud J H (1989) Psychosocial and neuropsychiatric aspects. *AIDS/HIV Infection: A Reference Guide for Nursing Professionals*, 145–168. Philadelphia: W B Saunders.

Fox R C, Aiken L H and Messikomer C M (1990) The culture of caring: AIDS and the nursing profession. *The Milbank Quarterly*, **68**(Suppl. 2), 226–255.

Gallagher R M (1990) AIDS: the fear of contagion. *Nursing Standard*, **4**, 19, 30–32.

George H (1988) Psychological aspects of AIDS. *Medicine International*, 2352–2356.

George R and Hart G (1989) The Bloomsbury response to HIV and AIDS. *Responding to the AIDS Challenge: A Comparative Study of Local AIDS Programmes in the United Kingdom*. London: Health Education Authority/Longman.

Hannon S (1990) Adaptable nursing care plan for AIDS patients at home. *AIDS Patient Care*, April, 23–30.

Hart G and Fitzpatrick R (1990) Gay men, social support and HIV disease: a study of social integration in the gay community. *AIDS Care* **2**, 2, 163–170.

Hay L (1988) *The AIDS Book: Creating a Positive Approach*. Santa Monica, California: Hay House

Jekot W F and Purdy D W (1993) Treating HIV/AIDS patients with anabolic steroids. *AIDS Patient Care*, **7**, 2, 68–74.

Jourard S M (1970) Living and dying. *American Journal of Nursing*, **70**, February, 269–275.

Kilbane M P J, O'Donnell F and McKnight A (1989) Preparing the way in Northern Ireland. *Responding to the AIDS Challenge: A Comparative Study of Local AIDS Programmes in the United Kingdom*. London: Health Education Authority/Longman.

King M B (1987) AIDS and the general practitioner: psycho-social issues. *Health Trends* **19**, 1–3.

King M B (1989) Prejudice and AIDS. *AIDS Care*, **1**, 2, 137–143.

Kobasa S C O (1990) AIDS and volunteer associations: perspectives on social and individual change. *The Milbank Quarterly*, **68**(Suppl. 2), 280–294.

Lande R (1988) The role of the GP in the care of people with HIV infection and AIDS. *AIDS: Models of Care*, London: King's Fund.

Lang C (1993) Positive steps. *Nursing Times*, **89**, 11, 54–56.

Librach S L (1988) Who's in control? What's in a family? *Journal of Palliative Care*, **4**, 4, 11–12.

Lynch L J (1977) *The Broken Heart: the Medical Consequences of Loneliness*. Sydney: Harper & Row.

Mansfield S J and Singh S (1989) The general practitioner and human immunodeficiency virus infection: an insight into patients' attitudes. *Journal of the Royal College of General Practitioners,* **39**, March, 104–105.

McCann K and Wadsworth E (1992) The role of informal carers in supporting gay men who have HIV related illness: what do they do and what are their needs? *AIDS Care,* **4**, 1, 25–34.

Meyer-Bahlburg H F L (1993) *Sexual disfunction in homosexual HIV+ men: associations with immune function, endocrine, neurologic and psychiatric factors.* 9th International Conference on AIDS, Berlin.

Miller D (1986) Psychology, AIDS, ARC and PGL. *The Management of AIDS Patients,* 131–150. London: Macmillan Press.

Miller J F (1985) Hope doesn't necessarily spring eternal – sometimes it has to be carefully mined and channeled. *American Journal of Nursing,* January, 23–25.

Milne R I G and Keene S M (1988) Are general practitioners ready to prevent the spread of HIV? *British Medical Journal,* **296**, 533–535.

Morgan M and Rogers J (1993) Intentional self-infection with HIV by long-term partners of HIV positive homosexual men. *AIDS Patient Care,* February, 10–15.

Mostert H A (1991) *Nurses in AIDS-care: their two challenges, separation and integration.* 2nd European Conference for Nurses in AIDS Care, Noordwijkerhout, The Netherlands.

O'Casey S (1980) *Three Plays: Juno and the Paycock.* London: Pan Books.

Ong E L C, Clarke K W, Dunbar E M and Mandal B K (1993) Health care of people with HIV: a survey of their views. *AIDS Patient Care,* **7**, 2, 98–101.

Peck K and Johnson S (1990) The role of nutrition in HIV infection: a report of the working party of the AIDS interest group of the BDA. *Journal of Human Nutrition and Dietetics,* **3**, 147–157.

Raveis V H and Seigel K (1991) The impact of care giving on informal or familial care givers. *AIDS Patient Care,* **5**, 1, 39–43.

Robinson D and Maynard A (1991) *HIV/AIDS and Social Care.* London: Universities of Hull and York, Scottish Home and Health Department and the Department of Health.

Roderick P and Stevens A (1989) Fighting the fire in Paddington and North Kensington. *Responding to the AIDS Challenge: a Comparative Study of Local AIDS Programmes in the United Kingdom.*

Schofferman J (1989) Care of the terminally ill person with AIDS. *International Ophthalmology Clinics,* **29**, 2, 127–130.

Sibbald B and Freeling P (1988) AIDS and the future general practitioner. *Journal of the Royal College of General Practitioners,* **38**, 500–502.

Sims R and Moss V (1991) *Terminal Care for People with AIDS.* London: Edward Arnold.

Singh S (1991) Primary care and HIV – rising to the challenge? *AIDS Patients – Current Clinical Issues.* London and Leeds: R C N.

Smith M (1989) *Ready, Willing and Able: a Study of Nurses Attitudes Towards People with AIDS.* London: Department of Health.

Sontag S (1988) *Aids and its Metaphors.* Harmondsworth: Penguin Books.

Stables T (1990) AIDS and gay men. *Journal of District Nursing,* April, 20–26.

Webb C (1985) *Sexuality, Nursing and Health.* Chichester: John Wiley and Sons.

White K (1989) Alternative therapies: counselling patients about questionable treatments. *AIDS Patient Care,* December, 12–14.

Wilkie P (1992) Particular issues in working with partners. *Reflective Helping in HIV and AIDS,* 253–260. Milton Keynes: Open University Press.

Worden J W (1983) *Grief Counselling and Grief Therapy.* London: Tavistock Publications.

Chapter 6
Sexuality and Disability
Michael Morgan

Introduction

Until comparatively recently, 'sexuality' and 'disability' were words which rarely appeared in the same book, and almost never in the same sentence. The existence of a sexual side to disability was not only unmentioned, it went unrecognised by many, and even ignored by those in a position to know. In fact, disability was often assumed to preclude sexual expression, and asexuality an inevitable consequence. To be disabled was to be sexually dead.

However, we are repeatedly assured that all that belongs to a bygone age, to the Neolithic period of mutual misunderstanding between able-bodied and disabled, or so at least we are told. In fact, these old prejudices, presumptions and social non-expectations show a remarkable resilience among broad swathes of the population, particularly at the more popular levels of public discourse (Smith and Jordan 1991).

Of course, it remains true that there has been a major upswing in attention given to the area of sexuality and disability over the past twenty years and a marked openness in discussion of sexual matters which has put the problem centre-stage in any overall debate on disability – where, indeed, it belongs. This attention is most usually expressed in writing, in a growing volume of studies on both sides of the Atlantic, but also, hearteningly, in the formation and operation of specific organisations designed to respond to these needs. Perhaps the only drawback is that, so far, this discussion has taken place within the realms of specialised knowledge, whether within medicine and paramedical practice or among the disabled themselves; it has not, as yet, begun to permeate public consciousness in any significant way.

Hence the purpose of the present chapter is to provide nurses with a general overview of the situation regarding sexuality and disability, both from the point of view of their immediate role as health care professionals and from the wider standpoint of their role as members of society.

History of Disabled Sexuality

The catalyst in the upsurge in intellectual interest in the area of sexuality and disability was the publication, in 1974, of K Heslinga's *Not Made of Stone*, a graphic and frank account of the mostly physical difficulties experienced by people with disabilities in expressing their sexuality, whether in terms of specific genital dysfunction or as a consequence of earlier physical ability. This was not in any way surprising, as Heslinga was a medical doctor and had based his analysis on studies carried out in The Netherlands and Scandinavia, but it did carry with it a number of assumptions regarding the nature of the problem that were to stick. First, it helped to define the 'problem' as a medical–physical one, as one primarily to do with the functioning (or rather, non-functioning) of the individual human body and this, in turn, promoted a 'how-to-do-it' sort of approach, with 'it' meaning coitus. Secondly, an associated point, it located the 'problem' as occurring within the bedroom, in the (marital) bed, so to speak. The wider social context, a no less critical area for the formation and maintenance of sexual relationships was, by comparison, ignored.

Unquestionably, however, Heslinga's original analysis opened up the entire area of sexuality and disability for renewed scholarly attention and a whole series of books, pamphlets and other material was produced, of which Comfort (1978) is a particularly well-known example within the UK, while a review and re-examination of Heslinga's original findings has been carried out by his former collaborators (Dechesne 1985).

In the US, a parallel upsurge in writing on sexuality and disability has developed into an almost academic sub-discipline. Many American universities carry out research programmes into sexuality and disability, such as at Berkeley, California. A particularly interesting feature of the American scene is that researchers there have indeed widened their discussions to include the principally social context within which sexual interaction takes place. Studies such as that by Robinault (1978) focus on developmental issues facing the disabled youngster from the 'pre-teens' onwards, as he or she attempts to form a sexual identity within the constraints imposed by disability. The 'interface' between disabled and able-bodied is further examined in Seegert (1989), while other studies more closely resemble the medical–physical orientation displayed in the UK (e.g. Neistadt and Freda 1987).

In summary, therefore, there has been a major, and effective, upswing of interest among researchers, both academic and vocational, in the area of sexuality and disability over the past twenty years. The resulting avalanche of material and information has helped to bring more sharply into focus both the nature of these problems and the possible means of dealing with them, whether through counselling or therapy or even, simply, through education. This approach is not without its criticisms, but nevertheless it does represent a significant (and highly welcome) shift away from the earlier position of blanket ignorance, when not only were these problems not discussed, they were not even deemed to exist in the first place.

Persons and Problems: Not One, but Many

The public mind knows well, or pretends to know, what a 'disabled person' looks like. A particularly common image is that of a robust, otherwise fit and healthy young man or woman in relatively full control of his or her life but for the fact of using a wheelchair. The image projected by Jon Voight in the film *Coming Home* – that of the paraplegic Vietnam War veteran – has become a cultural stereotype, it seems. For a (very) brief time disability became something glamorous, even sexy. But of course it could not last – and it did not. 'Macho wheelchair' became redundant as a phrase as soon as it was uttered.

The fact that paraplegics make up only a small proportion of people designated as 'the disabled' is, in consequence, overlooked. Thus the danger of using a single, collective noun to denote what is, in reality, a very wide range of life experiences must be obvious. People with disabilities differ from each other over an enormous range of variables.

First, and most obviously, they differ in basic medical condition – there are blind people, deaf people, people with speech difficulties, partially or completely paralysed people, people whose brain or nervous systems have been damaged through genetic defect, illness or accident, people disabled as a result of viral infection, such as polio, or AIDS – an immense range. But also, and just as obviously, they differ on almost every other significant variable known: in terms of sex, sexual preference, age, social class, education, race, ethnicity, religion, cultural background, morality and doubtless a few more.

This wide divergence in life experiences among people collectively designated as 'the disabled' is, however, sometimes overlooked. There are reasons, of course: social planners in the welfare, medical and nursing systems need to refer to a single, undifferentiated category of 'people with disabilities' in order to design and provide services. As well, having a disability in itself helps to make a common identity, at least in so far as being at the sharp end of social exclusion and prejudice creates one. A common dependence on the state and its medical, social security and welfare systems, and consequent close association with the often Byzantine workings of the welfare bureaucracy, helps create a common 'constituency of interest' among otherwise heterogeneous individuals.

However, this is only the 'official', public, face of disability, a world of shared concerns wherein 'people with disabilities' coalesce into a single collectivity to forward 'their' interests. Public roles are experienced collectively; but the private is experienced personally. In their private lives, widespread differences in life situations and experiences between people with disabilities re-asserts themselves – and what could be more private than sexuality?

Sexuality is what a person is. An almost total gulf divides, for instance, a middle-aged father-of-four paraplegic and a similarly disabled seventeen-year-old. A congenitally blind man or deaf woman may experience no difficulties whatsoever in the mechanics of the thing, but may well find a lack of opportunity to engage in sexual relationships to be their problem. Perhaps, then, we should think of the whole area of sexuality and disability as posing different kinds of problems for different kinds of individuals with different kinds of disabilities. Any discussion must therefore try to accommodate this basic divergence within a general analytical framework.

Broadly speaking, problems in sexuality and disability can be divided between physical problems and relational problems. 'Physical problems' refer to the 'mechanics' of sex. One thinks immediately of medical conditions which cause sexual dysfunction, such as certain muscular and neuromuscular diseases, spinal injuries of varying seriousness, etc., or even of those disabling conditions which interfere with, and sometimes make impossible, 'normal' sexual functioning, such as the more serious forms of spasticity, paralysis, etc.

'Relational problems', on the other hand, refers to difficulties experienced by people with disabilities in forming and sustaining sexual relationships. The problems experienced here are different in kind from the simply physical; in fact, a different reality. 'Problems' herein are psychological and, possibly primarily, social in character; that is, they refer to the *micropersonal* world of human interaction which the individual inhabits (Christians 1985). It need not necessarily be the disabled individual's 'problem' – at least in so far as 'problem' implies 'fault' – but may indeed have more to do with the reactions of others, from small-scale interaction where able-bodied unease gives rise to personal avoidance strategies, through to the full-blown sociological process of stigmatisation leading to outright rejection. This latter, alas, as we shall shortly see, seems at times inherent in general social conditioning.

In practice, of course, the two are inseparable: physical problems are most often experienced as relational problems. Sex, beyond onanism, is an inter-personal reality wherein human individuals interact with one another. Physical problems are related to *performance* and will initially register as relational problems: a disability-linked failure to achieve ejaculation will become translated as worries about being unable to satisfy one's partner, or even as reason to avoid a sexual relationship in the first place. In effect, the relational subsumes the physical as the major seat of problems and anxiety over sexuality and disability. This point is often overlooked – even by writers and professionals involved in the field of sexuality and disability.

A final point: much, if not most, of the anxieties, difficulties and worries experienced by people with disabilities in their sexual roles, and in their sexuality, are in no appreciable fashion different from those experienced by many others in today's society. Many of those in a similar position of social exclusion – the gay and lesbian communities, for example – will readily identify with the depiction of the issues of sexuality and disability presented here. As well, many of those living in the supposed 'mainstream' of society, those reading this perhaps, may well recognise at least some of the problems and dilemmas as their own.

The Physical Dimension

There exists already a voluminous, and ever-growing, literature concentrating on the physical side of sexuality and disability. It is not my intention to reproduce this here in detail, but rather to sketch in the general outlines of the area for those who wish for an overall picture. For a more detailed description, for instance of the precise effects of specific medical conditions, see especially Pons (1985) and Heslinga (1974).

The basic outlines of this area have already been touched upon. We can differentiate between direct and indirect effects of various disabling conditions on an individual's sexual functioning. Direct conditions cause *sexual dysfunction* – specific disruption of or damage to the body's reproductive system. Indirect conditions can have negative effects on sexual functioning but do not cause specific damage to the reproduction system *per se*.

Pons (1985) approaches his analysis of sexual problems and neurological injuries in terms of aspect, not condition. There is, first, the neuromuscular aspect – problems related to the nervous system, to the skeletal and muscular apparatus of the body, also known, according to Pons, as the instrumental aspect. Secondly, Pons writes of the genital aspect – problems related specifically to the sexual organs and their functioning, either at a neurophysiological, hormonal or gametogenical level. Thirdly, there is also a psycho-social aspect – psychological inhibitions governing physical activities, derived, at least in part, from wider social norms and attitudes.

Therefore, many people with disabilities suffer from conditions disrupting the functioning of their sexual organs (Pons' 'genital aspect'). Many more suffer disruption to their nervous, muscular and other systems which control sexual functioning (Pons' 'neuromuscular aspect'), or from wholly indirect causation such as paralysis, ataxia or spasticity, which can make such a strenuous, sheerly physical activity as sexual intercourse difficult (and sometimes impossible), while psychological anxiety and inhibition (Pons' 'psycho-social aspect') can cause an added dimension of problems.

The psycho-social aspect plays a major role in many conditions. Sex is usually considered an exclusively personal, pre-social activity, its workings a matter of biology, not society; but of course, social conditioning is ever-present in the prescription of sexual goals and behaviour just as it is in every other sort of behaviour. These goals and norms are then internalised by the individual as his or her own, and any inability to live up to them is experienced as a matter of purely personal shame and failure. Inhibition of physical sexual response closely follows and reinforces these psychological feelings of inadequacy in an ever-tightening circle.

Perhaps the most widespread social assumption concerns the primacy of intercourse as the defining sexual act: the belief that sexual intercourse *is* sex. But sexual intercourse raises numerous problems for many people with disabilities, ranging from the merely difficult (e.g., problems in movement and coordination) to those conditions which preclude intercourse altogether (e.g., impotence, vaginal disorders and, occasionally, incontinence).

Among these, impotence is an exclusively male problem. Females, by contrast, are said to be barren or infertile. This terminology, however, seems a little archaic. Better to say that problems in sexual intercourse are common to both men and women, even if the nature of those problems is different.

Male impotence can be defined as a failure to achieve erection and, in consequence, ejaculation. Without erection sexual intercourse leading to ejaculation is impossible. For the female the problems are different in kind, though no less traumatic in their effects. Vaginal secretion is a prerequisite for penetration without which sexual intercourse becomes difficult.

Direct medical intervention can often be of help here, usually pharmacologically but also, in the last resort, surgically. Erection in the male can, at times, be achieved through the administration of drugs such as Prostigmin, or a flaccid penis can be stiffened through the surgical insertion of various types of prostheses. Females may be supplied with various vaginal lubricants to restore functioning, at least in part. However, not only are there obvious limits to such intervention, but perhaps attention should focus more on people's assumptions and expectations regarding sex, particularly of the reductionism inherent in equating sexual intercourse with sex in general.

Sexual intercourse is often seen as the central act of sexuality, the big event around which everything else – intimacy, petting, love-making in its general, overall sense – is reduced to mere foreplay or otherwise deemed secondary. When sex was simply about procreation – that is, about reproduction in its most basic, biological sense as a means of procuring offspring – this definition held good. Nowadays, however, sex has largely ceased to be exclusively concerned with procreation and has, instead, come to be seen as a dispenser of a wider group of satisfactions. Sex may even be seen as a means to a further goal, no less cherished: intimacy. Individuals remain locked within barriers of self. Yet sex, and the attainment of intimacy with another that it entails, remains the core area of life where the barriers of self may be broken, or even transcended. Possibly in this, as much as in biology or chemistry, lies its modern meaning in human life.

Sex now opens up a whole range of sensuous possibilities and alternatives and is certainly not confined to a single activity. Sexual intercourse becomes one of many pursuits, rather than the one to which all else is subordinated. Feminist writer Andrea Dworkin made the point in a recent interview: 'If you haven't had sexual intercourse, why do you think you haven't had sex?'

Many people with disabilities experiencing problems in sexual intercourse – as well as many, similarly distressed, able-bodied people – would do well to reflect on this. It is a sad fact that people who experience such problems tend to see the successful attainment of intercourse as the one and only goal, and are prepared to put themselves through all manner of treatments, even surgery, in order to achieve this. As Pons says:

> Regardless of the type of prosthesis being considered, one must realise that such an enormous problem as impotence, with all of its physical, psychological and social implications, will not be solved simply by the insertion of a small rod. Good pre-operative counselling is needed in order to establish a differential organic/psychogenic diagnosis, and to offer the patient and his partner acceptable, alternative approaches to sexual activity.
>
> (Pons 1985, 81)

Therefore education, the dissemination of information on the development of alternative sexual practices, as well as a general re-orientation towards sex (through counselling, perhaps) could be as effective and satisfactory a solution as reliance on various aids, drugs or other gadgetry to 'restore' former prowess.

Incontinence is a major daily worry for many people with disabilities, just as it is, incidentally, for many able-bodied people. Problems in management of the body's waste products are the focus of perhaps the most stringent of social taboos: incontinence remains a 'hidden disability' which is often a source of much misery and anxiety. In terms of sexuality and disability the effect can be quite devastating. Among people with disabilities incontinence can be a major inhibitor of sexual desire: genitals have a dual function, both as sexual organs and as conduits for the expelling of urine. The anus is also a highly sexually charged zone. Personal hygiene is paramount. Permanent catheterisation or living with a stoma operation produces an altered body image, sometimes a re-ordering of bodily parts, and one that can be particularly difficult to handle in sexual situations. Also, in this context, menstruation can be a difficult time, especially for the wheelchair-bound female (Boylan 1991). There are, moreover, no easy solutions. Many field-workers in the area of sexuality and disability report the prevalence of incontinence as a major problem, with most effort going into counselling and advice on personal management and control. The original attraction and feeling, leading to mutual trust, established between sexual partners should be strong enough to cope with this and other, merely physical, problems. This is only to repeat what has been said before: that problems in sexuality and disability, whether physical or otherwise, always present themselves as relational problems and are, as often as not, resolved at this level as well.

Relationships

Sex is perhaps our strongest link with the animal world around us from which we developed, a world of rank physicality. Yet sex is also the site of the most elaborate social rituals and rule-governed behaviours known. Our terminology reflects this divide: sex and sexuality. Sex may be taken to refer simply to the physical act, or acts, involved. Sexuality, however, encompasses sexual interaction, a different reality. In particular it refers to the micro-personal world of daily contact. This is where the rituals of sexuality are performed: where strangers become friends who (may) become lovers. This, too, is the most important area in any overall discussion of disabled sexuality; yet oddly enough, it also seems to be comparatively ignored in the literature.

People with disabilities tend to be excluded from the micropersonal world wherein initial sexual contact is usually made. They may also, as a direct consequence of this exclusion, suffer repeated – and highly damaging – blows to their inner concept of self and self-esteem, a critical resource for effective sexuality.

Adolescents with Disabilities

Sexual interaction is best thought of as a game, albeit a serious one. It is a 'game' whose rules and governing principles are laid down during adolescence, the 'dangerous bend' between childhood and adulthood when the experience of puberty transforms every aspect of individual existence and identity (Taylor 1991). 'Normal' adolescence is universally a period of turmoil and stress: the secure world of childhood existence is left behind as a new search for adult identity begins.

Adolescence is seen as a rite of passage into adult existence, troublesome, arduous even, but above all natural – a necessary grounding in the realities of life faced by every individual. It is where the rules governing male/female interaction – or erotic grammar – are first laid down. Learning about sex is much more than understanding the biology of reproduction: what does what and why? The most important things to know are not taught – at least, not formally. These are the things which are 'picked up' through immersion in peer-group culture, providing a rudimentary sexual skills training: seeking out the other, recognising sexual signals and body language, conversational abilities (is referred to in adolescent parlance as 'chatting up'). The peer group is the most important source of authority over the individual adolescent's behaviour. It 'rewards' those who model themselves most closely on group norms and 'punishes' those who do not through the dispensation of status (in adolescent parlance, 'street cred'); and status is the key to sexual success in the teenage years (Anderson and Clarke 1982).

For the adolescent with disabilities even entry into a peer group may be difficult. While childhood friendships make no distinction between disabled and able-bodied companions (save that, perhaps, of curiosity) adolescence brings the distinction between disabled and able-bodied to the fore. Many earlier friendships come to a bad end as the influence of the peer group takes over – the disabled teenager is desperate not to be excluded, the able-bodied friend is torn between loyalty to his or her 'chum' and the pressures of the new. Underlying this, of course, is the draw of sexuality itself. Not many friendships survive that.

Sometimes the teenager with disabilities is marginalised within the group, allowed to participate in most group activities, which now include going to dances, drinking in pubs, etc., but who is quietly but firmly excluded from the core activity around which the peer group is formed: sexual interaction. If he or she attempts to challenge this unspoken, indeed largely unacknowledged, rule, they will soon discover that there are limits to their acceptance within the group, and those limits are set very firmly around situations of ritualised sexual interaction. Any number of anecdotes can illustrate this. A young girl in a wheelchair is employed in the Civil Service. She is immediately befriended by her able-bodied peers and enters into the collective life of the place, sharing with her friends in all social activities. All except one, that is. When it comes to going to dances, or otherwise engaging in purposeful male–female interaction, she finds herself excluded, usually subtly but backed up with positive discouragement if necessary. In her pioneering study of the psychological consequences of disability, Beatrice Wright observed that exclusion from sexual situations had been a major, debilitating, feature of the adolescence of many people with disabilities. She wrote:

> These accounts reveal a deep and sometimes overwhelming loneliness. These young people were lonely not because of lack of friendship, but because they could not share in boy–girl relationships.
>
> (Wright 1960, 189)

One way of trying to offset this 'normal' tendency to exclude was the formation of the PHAB clubs in the early 1970s. PHAB (Physically Handicapped and Able-Bodied) was designed as a network of youth clubs 'mixing' disabled and able-bodied teenagers together, the idea being that full integration between the two groups within a club setting would lead to a similar integration within the wider social environment. Although the PHAB philosophy may not have been explicitly designed with a 'sexual' motive in mind, the overall aim of social integration which PHAB sought to achieve would none the less also imply sexual integration. But has it worked? The short answer is 'no'. Its charity status marks it off as a 'special' group: hence, for those with 'street cred', as something to be avoided. Even within the club setting rival peer groups tend to form. One observer at a PHAB disco reported the teenagers with disabilities congregating at one end of the hall, and the able-bodied teenagers at the other. Adolescence, therefore, continues to be a rough time for teenagers with disabilities, the first experience of what it means to be disabled in an able-bodied world.

Adults with Disabilities

At the end of adolescence lies adulthood. If adolescence is a transition state, then adulthood is supposedly the finished state of sexual maturity. The experience of disability can, however, drastically alter an individual's development. Baldly stated, lack of opportunity is the single most important problem faced by many adults with disabilities in expressing their sexuality. They may know very well *what* to do, and may not even be unduly concerned at any physical problem in doing it, but it is finding someone to do it *with* that constitutes the real problem. Knowing what to do is not enough.

Reasons for the lack of sexual opportunities among people with disabilities are primarily *external*, having most to do with the status and perceived role of people with disabilities within society (Porter 1987). However, the situation may in turn have negative consequences for *internal* psychological health, creating loss of self-esteem and failure in self-confidence. And these are vital attributes when it comes to engaging in effective sexual interaction.

Disability, Self and Social Exclusion

The micropersonal world refers to the border zone between friendship and acquaintance wherein the rituals of sexuality are performed, the 'meeting ground' where strangers become friends, become lovers – as the case may be. It encompasses much of the daily social routine common to both sexes: going to pubs, clubs and dances. It is ever present in the world of work, an important area for male–female interaction and initial sexual contact.

People with disabilities, however, tend to be excluded from the micropersonal world for a number of reasons. First, there are marked differences in disabled life-style which serve to increase isolation, exclusion and barriers to integration. Many people with disabilities are poor, dependent on state benefits of various kinds for their income (Dalley 1991). There are other, no less damaging, consequences. Finding suitable independent accommodation is a major problem for people with disabilities, who are often forced to remain in their parental home; without privacy, without control and often under conditions of asexuality. Residential homes, sometimes the only alternative, offer little improvement (if not worse). Suitable transport, or rather the lack of it, is another major problem despite the undoubted success of the 'Motability' car-ownership scheme. Also to be considered here is the admittedly well-known problem of access to public buildings: pubs, restaurants, theatres, and the like. The key importance of employment has already been stressed. However, it has been estimated that of the 2·6 million people with disabilities of working age in the UK, only a third are in employment. Even here 'employment' can often mean home-based work, for instance on a computer keyboard, which is usually something considerably less than full immersion in the social and interpersonal environment of the workplace that makes 'work' such an important social activity in the first place. In all, therefore, we can say that there are major differences in life-style between people with disabilities and their able-bodied counterparts, and these differences combine to reinforce the exclusion of people with disabilities from the micropersonal environment. A related point is that the sort of social contact that people with disabilities *do* participate in is not normally conducive to sexual interaction. Day-centres are notorious for providing no sex education of any kind, and ignoring any mention of sexuality at all among their 'clients' (Barnes 1990), nor does the sort of charity evening organised by various voluntary groups offer much scope for erotic negotiations. One partial exception, oddly enough, remains that of organised group holidays, particularly trips abroad. Many relationships have been formed on holiday, and have lasted the course – proof, if it was needed, that once access to a micropersonal environment is made the rest, so to speak, follows naturally.

The second reason for the exclusion of people with disabilities from the micropersonal world is the operation of *stigmatisation* – a process of social exclusion aimed at those deviant from the 'norm'. Without doubt the key area where stigmatisation occurs at its most virulent remains that of sexual interaction. Erving Goffman provided a succinct example when he recounted how one disabled individual (a blind girl) chanced to overhear one of her (able-bodied) companions say to his companion: 'Obviously, I like Diana very much, but I would never go out with a blind girl' (Goffman 1968, 46). It is the absolute quality of that statement that jars – 'I would *never* go out with a blind girl'. This is not simply prejudice on the part of a few ideologically unreconstructed individuals (although, of course, it can be just that, too). Clearly, there is something of general sociological significance going on. Stigmatisation against the disabled may be related to a societal need to preserve the whole by erecting barriers against those so clearly, if innocently, in transgression of the 'norms' upon which it is based. At a deeper, anthropological, level, stigmatisation against the disabled may be considered functional to society in narrowing down the reproductive chances for 'deviant' people with disabilities. Quite possibly, the exclusion of people with disabilities from the sexual arena may have had its origins in biological – even genetic – imperatives, as a form of naturally occurring eugenics, as it were. Other, probably more direct, influences include the continuing lack of economic power among people with disabilities and their (consequent?) low status. Perhaps the most important, however, is their perceived inability to fulfil a parental role within a new family structure. Sexual interaction is a serious business, a 'game' in many ways, but always with the underlying aim of mate selection (and family formation) in mind. Because of this, sexual interaction demands strict conformity from all those wishing to enter as a 'player'. An individual's potential as possible co-parent remains the deciding factor in mate selection, but under such conditions people with disabilities may find themselves excluded even from consideration as a potential partner. Also in this context, marriages between able-bodied and disabled partners are frequently frowned upon. The able-bodied prospective partner often receives a stern warning, usually from parents, in terms of 'throwing your life away' should the marriage go through.

Disability and the Inner Self

What makes a person attractive to others is his or her inner self – what used to be called strength of character – rather than mere external appearance. But the self is itself nourished on self-esteem or self-value – the belief in oneself that underlies how the individual asserts his or her presence and projects his or her personality. Without this basic belief in oneself it becomes difficult to even approach someone, let alone try to establish a sexual relationship with them.

Lack of self-esteem is a major, perhaps *the* major problem among people with disabilities of all age groups. Many psychological studies report the development of a basically passive, isolative orientation to interpersonal interaction among adolescents with disabilities (Harper and Richman 1978). These experiences of psychological withdrawal also extend far into adulthood, making all kinds of meaningful interaction difficult. Prosser (1992) cites research, in particular that of Vamos (1990) who reported loss of self-esteem and value among women whose hands had been disfigured as a result of rheumatoid arthritis, and had trouble coming to terms with the resulting alteration in body-image.

Lack of self-esteem may come, in the first place, from the general negativity inherent in the disabled lifestyle. Disability is pathological: a 'problem' for medical services, nursing staff, potential employers, housing managers, etc. These negative experiences are often internalised psychologically by people with disabilities in terms of 'being a burden' on others, or of being somehow 'less than normal'. In this way negative experiences become negative expectations. Being convinced of their own inadequacies, many people with disabilities fail to achieve that special sense of confidence in themselves that is a prerequisite for effective sexual interaction. Some foreclose on the sexual side of life altogether, and sink into a twilight world of permanent childhood and asexuality. They become the passive 'family cripple' stereotype, wearing special clothes, or may develop a 'Quasimodo complex' – where even the possibility of sexual awareness is routinely, and aggressively, denied. The importance of the lack of self-esteem among people with disabilities as the major factor in their lack of sexual interaction was well recognised by Dechesne:

> What consequences do various disabilities carry for the sense of self-value, and subsequently for the sexuality and relationships of handicapped people?
>
> (Dechesne, 1985, 128)

Self-esteem is an internal quality that is essentially responsive to the actions of others. Many people with disabilities face everyday situations not knowing exactly how to respond to others, and also many others find it difficult to respond to *them*. There may be no 'script', or commonly agreed stock of knowledge to deal with such social interactions. Instead, recourse is made to stereotypes, and these stereotypes can often be negative. People with disabilities are often patronised in situations of interpersonal communication – the *Does He Take Sugar?* syndrome. Being patronised carries with it implied inferiority. As such it can be a painful blow to self-esteem (Prosser 1992).

In a recent interview disabled scientist and author Professor Stephen Hawking remarked that he chose to laugh at people who patronised him, to make light of it (and thus dismiss it as of no consequence). This is, on the face of it, a healthy response. However, it must be remembered that Hawking does so from an already secure position, as a world-ranking astrophysicist and best-selling author. Many, perhaps most, people with disabilities do not attain the same sort of external success in life and so may not develop that special sense of self-worth needed to be able to 'laugh if off'. For many, the experience of being patronised continues to be a painful blow to self-esteem precisely because there was not much there in the first place.

We have, so far, been addressing the major problem area faced by people with disabilities in expressing their sexuality, that of forming sexual relationships. There is, however, an important exception to this: people with disabilities who experience problems in existing relationships. These are, usually, people who acquire what is termed a late-onset disability, individuals who may already have reached the state of adulthood and whose sexual status is (or has previously been) considered 'normal'. They may already be in a more or less stable long-term relationship (possibly with children). One thinks immediately, for example, of people who have suffered a disabling accident at work or who have become paralysed as the result of a car crash. Then again, there will be people who acquire a debilitating neurological disease, such as MS or Parkinson's, in later life, or even those with a progressive genetic disorder such as Friedreich's ataxia, who may enter into a long-term relationship at an early stage yet find the increasing level of disability more of a strain as the years progress.

One much-cherished and widespread myth is that, whenever disability intervenes in a relationship in this way, it is the duty of the able-bodied partner to remain steadfast and loyal – 'in sickness and in health, till death do us part'. Society rewards such unselfish devotion on the part of the healthy partner by according them heroic status: partners who remain are often sanctified as latter-day saints while, in contrast, those who go are as often pilloried as unfeeling egotists, or worse. The reality is, however, that a high proportion of such relationships, alas, tend to crack open under the strain. Such break-ups also tend to be emotionally messy. The able-bodied former partner often experiences guilt and shame, while the disabled former partner often feels betrayed. The frequency of such break-ups is itself testament to the fact that coping with disability imposes great strain on the relationship.

All sexual relationships are based on a underlying power balance whose roots lie in the nature of the original sexual 'contract' between the two people involved. The nature of any relationship, frankly, continues to be determined largely by the sexual power of each respective individual within it. The effect of trauma caused by sudden or late-onset disability may be such as to reverse the 'normal' roles and polarities within a relationship, causing enormous strain. Moreover, as people continue to be conditioned into the social expectations outlined above, their immediate response will be one of denial that any such problem exists, coupled with private shame at the realisation that it does. In this way professional help – counselling, psycho-sexual therapy – will not be sought until, of course, it is too late. Some people just cannot come to terms with the sudden loss in sexual ability that disability may bring. PC Philip Olds, a policeman paralysed in a gun attack, revealed his inner angst on camera to a visiting BBC documentary team in *The Visit*. Unable to come to terms with the loss of sexual power, Olds led an increasingly desperate quest for a 'miracle-cure' – eventually shooting himself when he reached the end of his tether. An extreme case, maybe, but one which nevertheless highlights the degree of emotional trauma in coping with sudden disability and loss of sexual power that is its consequence.

Conclusion: What is to be Done?

What *should* be done must be qualified by what *can* be done. Sexual interaction will always involve discrimination. Ideologies of equal access hold no influence here. There is a danger in raising expectations to unrealistic levels. Life will continue to be rough for people with disabilities, no matter how enlightened society becomes. We have disposed of one stereotype (the asexual 'family cripple') but we must be careful not to create another (the 'wheelchair raver').

Education, and the dissemination of information on all aspects of sexuality and disability, continues to play the major role both for academics and for voluntary organisations such as SPOD (the association to aid the Sexual and Personal relationships of people with a Disability) or SIA (Spinal Injuries Association).

Sex counselling has become a major growth industry in recent years, in both state and voluntary sectors. DISCERN is a Nottingham-based organisation providing counselling for people with disabilities experiencing problems, most usually in existing relationships. Yet counselling only provides a partial answer. It may help to 'work through' sexual problems within a counselling session (certainly in the sense of giving legitimacy to unvoiced worries) but is rarely designed to lead to remedial action.

The use of surrogate therapy – where the counsellor enters into direct sexual relations with his/her client – has, from time to time, been mooted as a possible course of action in the UK, but has not met with widespread approval (Davies 1988). There are the usual objections; that surrogacy shades into prostitution, or that it offers sex without any emotional involvement on the part of the therapist. These objections are redoubled when it comes to people with disabilities, who are often held to be especially emotionally vulnerable and so at risk. In The Netherlands, however, surrogacy has been well established for some years. *Stichting Alternatieve Relatiebemiddeling* (SAR) operate throughout Holland. They argue that their service does not pretend to be anything other than a boost to self-confidence and self-esteem for people with disabilities, a sort of sexual first-aid. However, surrogacy is a political hot potato in the UK and is likely to remain so for the foreseeable future.

Perhaps the catalyst for change in sexuality and disability might be an indirect one. The major problem faced by people with disabilities is a lack of sexual opportunities in everyday life, the main reasons being that people with disabilities tend to be excluded from the micropersonal environment wherein sexual interaction takes place. Measures of general social integration for people with disabilities may well prove a more far-reaching reform than anything aimed specifically at sexuality and disability in particular (Barnes 1992). Employment is a vital area for reform, bringing people with disabilities within one of the most important micropersonal environments for sexual interaction. The provision of accessible housing, allowing people with disabilities the freedom to lead independent lives, is another. Also to be included is the question of accessible transport provision. And finally, of course, there is the well-known problem of physical access to public places – restaurants, cinemas, pubs, etc.

The overall problem, then, is that people with disabilities have been marginalised into the backwaters of social life, where opportunities for sexual interaction are limited and difficult. This lack of opportunity, in turn, leads to profound psychological and social malaise and sexual interaction remains a problem area. Most people with disabilities and their organisations, including the self-styled 'Disability Movement', argue that the best means of countering this historical marginalisation is by renewed integration of people with disabilities at all levels of society. This will, of course, have important consequences. Sexuality and disability raise problems which may be best resolved, in the long term, at this more general level of the integration of people with disabilities within society.

References

Anderson E and Clarke L (1982) *Disability and Adolescence*. London: Methuen.
Barnes C (1990) *Cabbage Syndrome: The Social Construction of Dependency*. London: Falmer Press.
Barnes C (1992) *Disabled People and Discrimination in Britain: A Case for Anti-Discrimination Legislation*. London: Hurst & Co. Ltd.
Boylan C (1991) *Women and Disability*. London: Zed Books.
Christians M (1985) We do it normally, just like other people. In Dechesne, B H H, Pons, C and Schellen A M C M *Sexuality and Handicap*, 183–218. London: Woodhead Faulkner Ltd.
Comfort A (1978) *Sexual Consequences of Disability*. New York: Stickley.
Dalley G (1991) *Disability and Social Policy*. London: Policy Studies Institute.
Davies M (1988) Sex therapy with people with a physical disability. In Cole M and Dryden W (eds) *Sex Therapy in Britain*. Milton Keynes: Open University Press.
Dechesne B H H (1985) On the road to partnership. In Dechesne, B H H, Pons, C and Schellen A M C M (eds) *Sexuality and Handicap*, 123–143. London: Woodhead Faulkner Ltd.
Goffman E (1968) *Stigma: Notes on the Management of Spoiled Identity*. Harmondsworth: Penguin.
Harper D C and Richman L C (1978) Personality profiles of physically impaired adolescents. *Journal of Clinical Psychology, 43*, 3, 636–642.
Heslinga K (1974) *Not Made of Stone: The Sexual Problems of Handicapped People*. Leyden: Noordhoff International Publishing.
Neistadt M E and Freda M (1987) *Choices: Guide to Sex Counseling with Physically Disabled Adults*. New York: Praeger.
Pons C (1985) Sexual problems and neurological injuries. In Dechesne B H H, Pons C and Schellen A M C M (eds) *Sexuality and Handicap*, 49–64. London: Woodhead Faulkner Ltd.
Porter M (1987) *Sexuality and People with Physical Disabilities*. Geneva: World Health Organization.

Prosser G (1992) Psychological issues when others mediate your life. In Jones P R and Crowley-Bainton T (eds) *Psychology and Physical Disability* (special edition of *Educational and Child Psychology*, **9**, 1).

Robinault I P (1978) *Sex, Society and the Disabled: A Developmental Inquiry into Roles, Reactions and Responsibilities*. London: Harper & Row.

Seegert B (1989) *Nasty Girls, Thugs and Humans Like Us: Social Relationships between Severely Disabled and Non Disabled Students in High School*. New York: P H Brookes.

Smith S and Jordan A (1991) *Disability: What the Papers Say . . . and Don't Say*. London: Spastics Society.

Taylor D (1991) On becoming an adult. In *Choices: Transition to Adult Life for People with Genetic Disorders*. Oxford: Genetic Interest Group.

Vamos M (1990) Body image in rheumatoid arthritis: the relevance of hand appearance to desire for surgery. *British Journal of Medical Psychology*, **63**, 3, 267–277.

Wright B A (1960) *Physical Disability: A Psychological Approach*. New York: Harper.

Chapter 7
Mental Health and Sexuality
Kath Ferguson

Introduction

Sexuality affects all aspects of life and is intimately tied up with a person's mental health. Kuczynski emphasises that sexuality encompasses much more than just the physical act of sex, but also involves a person's self-image and self-esteem, their needs for relationships and love, and their masculine and feminine self-image (Kuczynski 1980). Issues related to sex and gender appear to play an important part in the aetiology of mental health problems. Likewise a breakdown in mental health and indeed some aspects of psychiatric treatment and care may have a detrimental effect on a person's sense of self and sexual relations. Clearly then, a consideration of a patient's sexuality is an important part of mental health care.

A review of the literature explores some of the many ways in which sexuality and mental health are linked, and the implications for nursing care. An examination of the incidence of mental health problems according to gender reveals a higher susceptibility to mental breakdown in women, particularly neurosis, depression and eating disorders. The influence of underlying social, political and economic factors and biological factors is considered as well as possible factors which have been largely ignored in traditional psychiatric treatment.

The close relationship between sexual dysfunction and mental health is explored. Any interference with a person's sexual sense of self is likely to cause considerable distress. In addition, mental health problems themselves may have a negative impact on a person's sexuality. A number of issues relating to sexuality and the psychiatric system are considered. Psychiatry has historically occupied a controlling or regulatory function in relation to sexuality – some of the ethical issues are explored. Issues of sexual harassment and abuse within the mental health setting are discussed.

Sexuality is also considered in relation to psychiatric nursing itself. Although this branch of nursing attracts more men a division of labour by gender is apparent, reflecting divisions in society as a whole. In the final section, in an attempt to draw together and apply the findings from the literature, a case example of a woman suffering from depression is explored in detail, identifying her potential needs in relation to sexuality, goals for care and nursing interventions. Sexuality seems to touch on so many aspects of mental health nursing, and consequently the literature is potentially vast, so it has been necessary in several instances to refer the reader to more specialist sources.

Mental Health and Sexuality

The Incidence of Mental Health Problems According to Gender

All the data on rates of mental illness in the West seem to suggest that women are more susceptible to mental health problems than men. Women are more likely to be referred to a psychologist, psychiatrist or therapist (Briscoe 1982) and are more likely to receive psychiatric treatment in hospital. In 1986, 482 women per 100,000 population were admitted to psychiatric units compared with 364 men (Russo 1990). Community studies, too, reveal that women suffer more emotional distress, much of which is undiagnosed (Huppert, Roth and Gove 1986, Blaxter 1987).

Women are twice as likely as men to be prescribed psychotropic drugs (Cooperstock 1976). In 1984, 21 million people in the UK were on tranquillisers or sedatives, and of these 14 million were women (Melville 1984). Surprisingly, the incidence of mental illness is reversed in childhood, with boys showing a higher incidence of behaviour disorders, language and perceptual disorders, infantile autism and drug abuse (Gomez 1991).

Types of Mental Health Problems According to Gender

The research also shows major differences in presentation of symptoms according to gender. Women are significantly more likely to suffer from neurosis and depression. A national survey of morbidity in general practices revealed that women consult their GP more often for depression and anxiety, the ratios being three women to one man and two-and-a-half women to one man respectively (Royal College of General Practitioners 1986). Woman are also three times as likely to attempt suicide or to mutilate themselves (Gomez 1991), and 10 to 20 times more likely to suffer from eating disorders (Duker and Slade 1988).

Meanwhile, men are more likely to suffer from alcoholism, psychopathy, mania, drug dependence and sexual deviance (Gomez 1991). They are also more likely to commit suicide, and to use violent means to do so (Garai 1970). While rates of schizophrenia are similar for men and women, men tend to show poorer adjustment and to be more difficult to deal with (Salokangas

1983, Gomez 1991). Ninety per cent of homeless people sleeping out are men, and this group has a high incidence of schizophrenia, alcoholism and personality problems (Gomez 1991).

While women are more likely to be diagnosed as mentally ill, men are more likely to be convicted of criminal offences. In 1986, in England, 36,743 men were in prison compared with only 1,229 women, and 1,376 men were in special hospitals compared with 337 women (Home Office 1986).

The fact that women tend to live longer, and that dementia strikes particularly in the older age groups, contributes to women's over-representation in in-patient statistics. In 1985, 58 per cent of admissions to mental illness units were women, but of those over 75 years 67 per cent were female, and of those over 90 years 80 per cent were female (Office of Health Economics 1987).

Biological or Social Explanations?

The notion of women being psychologically defective or inferior as a result of their reproductive system was particularly prominent in Victorian times (Showalter 1985), but is still around today. However, there is growing evidence to suggest that the idea that genetic factors or female hormones may account for gender differences is too simplistic (e.g. Rose, Lewontin and Kamin 1984).

Ussher (1991) suggests that pre-menstrual syndrome (PMS), post-natal depression (PND) and the menopause have all been used incorrectly to support biological theories of mental illness and to label women as 'out of control, unbalanced and unpredictable'. PMS is a relatively recently recognised 'disorder' which Birke (1986) attributes to progesterone imbalance. It has been associated with a myriad of symptoms including anxiety, tiredness, hostility, irritability, emotional lability, palpitations and reduced libido. PMS has also been linked with increased chance of psychiatric admission (Luggin et al 1984), murder (Hey 1985) and suicide (Mandell and Mandell 1969). However, research has shown that objective links between mood and the menstrual cycle are less clear (e.g. Sommer 1973). Depression is also well known as the commonest psychological side-effect associated with oral contraceptives, but work by Fleming and Seager (1978) showed there was no difference in the incidence of depression among women on 'the pill' compared to a matched control group. More important pre-disposing factors were age, personality and employment situation.

PND has also been implicated in the biology/environment debate. Dalton (1980) suggests that as many as one in ten women are depressed enough following childbirth to require medical help. However, there is no clear evidence that hormones are solely responsible. Severe psychiatric disorder appears to be more common where the woman has experienced difficulties during pregnancy and birth (Asch and Rubin 1974), suggesting that social and psychological factors must play some part. Ussher (1991) argues that there is no conclusive evidence for hormonal aetiology, and that depression following childbirth is natural, due to grieving for the 'lost-self', tiredness, lack of support and adjusting to a new role.

The menopause has been associated with a plethora of physical and psychological ailments including depression. La Rococco and Polit (1980), however, point out that the only symptom consistently identified with the menopause is vasomotor instability leading to hot flushes and profuse perspiration. Miles (1991) refers to the medicalisation of the menopause (which has been described in the USA as 'oestrogen deficiency disease!'), and argues that the location of psychological problems in the individual fails to take account of the impact of the social structure on middle-aged women.

Cross-cultural studies indicate a higher incidence of all mental illness, including depression in some countries, e.g. India and Uganda, which may be explained by environmental differences (Gomez 1991). Gordon and Ledray (1985) raise questions about the methodology of some of the studies on gender differences in relation to response bias, bias in sampling and lack of controls.

It seems, therefore, that biological factors alone cannot account for the extent of the differences in susceptibility of men and women to mental health problems, or why some women are affected and not others.

Gender Differences in Mental Health Problems – an Analysis of the Social Factors

An examination of the social factors believed to account for the different rates and types of mental health problems experienced by men and women reveals a highly complex picture. Part of the explanation may lie in the different characteristics and behaviours expected of males and females. Sex role stereotypes are influential from an early age and affect the way men and women behave and also how others perceive them. While boys are expected to be competitive, dominant, active, self-reliant and high achievers, girls are encouraged to be nurturing, responsible, submissive, gentle and obedient. For girls, pregnancy and motherhood are expected to form the 'core of their being', anything else being seen as peripheral (Walker 1990).

Different socialisation may mean that women more readily admit to emotional distress and are more likely to seek psychiatric help (Briscoe 1982). Community studies, however, suggest that women are in fact less likely to come forward for treatment than expected (Goldberg and Huxley 1980). Similar problems may present differently in men and women due to different expectations of how they should behave. It may be that women are socialised to turn anger inwards, leading to high rates of depression. Men, in contrast, are encouraged to express their anger outwardly, and hence show a higher incidence of violence, suicide, anti-social behaviour and alcoholism (Gomez 1991). Bibb and Chambless (1988) suggest that many men deal with agoraphobia by drinking heavily, and therefore present with an alcohol problem.

The idea that women are inherently more unstable is not a new one. Indeed, terms such as 'neurotic' and 'hysterical' are words which are invariably associated with females in our society. Gomez (1991) questions whether doctors may be reluctant to label men as 'neurotic', and Walker (1990) suggests that women may be more likely to receive a psychiatric diagnosis for a non-specific problem. As Webb (1992) points out, mental health professionals are likely to share cultural expectations of appropriate behaviour for men and women, which influence the way we assess patients, decide on goals and what behaviour is seen as abnormal.

There is evidence to suggest that the stereotypical characteristics and behaviour of women are seen as less mentally healthy. Broverman et al (1970) asked psychologists, psychiatrists and social workers to describe the characteristics of a mature, socially competent male, female and adult (sex unspecified). It was found that the traits ascribed to a healthy male related more closely to descriptions of a healthy adult. Conceptions of a healthy woman, in contrast, i.e. submissive, passive, dependent, more emotional, differed significantly. While women are expected to conform to social norms, typical female characteristics are considered generally less desirable and healthy, raising questions about how women are expected to achieve mental health. Bem (1974), in an attempt to move away from a dichotomous conceptualisation of gender, developed the Bem Sex Role Inventory. Subjects were asked to rate themselves on a seven-point scale indicating how well they matched with 20 typically male and 20 typically female characteristics, and from this an 'androgyny score' was given. Those subjects with a high androgyny score, i.e. a high level of both male and female traits, were rated as having better psychological health in terms of self-esteem, spontaneity, self-acceptance and capacity for intimate relations. Those with lower self-esteem tended to have high feminine or low masculine and feminine typing (Miles 1991).

Society imposes expectations not only about how women should *be* but also about how they should *look*, which may be a source of stress. The development of anorexia in young women has been linked with current cultural attitudes favouring slimness (Bruch 1974) and its associations in the media with 'success, wealth, love, sexuality and happiness' (Orbach 1976). Some feminists regard anorexia as a protest against the way women are regarded as ornamental objects in society (Brumberg 1988). Others have argued that anorexia represents an attempt to avoid adulthood and the pressures arising from the girl's emergent sexuality. It is likely that all these theories only represent a part of the picture. (For a fuller discussion of the issues see Duker and Slade 1988.)

It appears, then, that by conforming to gender appropriate behaviour women are at risk of being diagnosed as mentally ill. Ussher (1991) argues further, however, that those women who have dared to deviate from prescribed female roles (e.g. witches, wise women, suffragettes) have been scapegoated in the past and today are also at risk of being diagnosed as 'mad'. She suggests that this treatment of women who deviate is a reflection of a misogynist society and a means of controlling and silencing those who threaten the social order. It seems, therefore, that women are in a no-win situation: damned if they do conform to sex-role stereotypes and damned if they don't!

Further light can be thrown on gender difference in mental health by considering the different roles occupied by men and women in society, and the value placed on these roles. It appears from the research that men fare better than women in marriage, in terms of psychological health. While married men have better mental health than single men, single women who have never been married have fewer psychiatric symptoms than any other group (Gove and Tudor 1972). As a group, males are more likely to commit suicide, but those most at risk are single, widowed or divorced men (Gomez 1991).

It is likely that within a traditional marriage, men's domestic, physical and emotional needs are better catered for than women's. In her work with subjects diagnosed as 'neurotic', Miles (1988) found that only 24 out of 65 women named their husband as their major confidante, many claiming that he failed to appreciate their emotional needs or provide support, whereas of the 20 men, 17 named their wives as a major confidante. Lack of a supportive relationship has been identified as a major risk factor in the onset of depression (Brown and Harris 1978).

Having children also seems to be a potential source of stress to women. High rates of depression are reported among women with young children, especially where the children have behavioural or health difficulties (McBride 1988). Brown and Harris (1978), too, identified women with young children as being at high risk of depression. Other risk factors were being working-class, lack of paid employment outside the home, absence of a close, confiding relationship and losing their mother as a child. Around 50 per cent of the women had experienced recent severe life events associated especially with loss, compared with 19 per cent of a control group. Ongoing major difficulties such as financial hardship and housing problems were more common in depressed women.

Research on the effects of employment on the health of women is particularly difficult to unravel. Housework is described by Oakley (1974) as depressing and unrewarding. Women are often isolated, with little structure to their lives, and the work is afforded low status in society, thus leading to low self-esteem, lack of confidence and dissatisfaction. Women may, however, experience guilt for feeling unfulfilled by the domestic and maternal role for which they have been socialised (Sharpe 1984).

In general, the evidence seems to suggest that women benefit psychologically from paid employment. Hibbard and Pope (1985) point out that employment may be beneficial in providing social contacts, giving independence, raising self-esteem, providing a routine and enabling people to feel as if they are contributing to society. Unemployment studies have revealed the damaging effects of not working on men's psychological health (Platt and Dyer 1987), with higher rates of depression, suicide and parasuicide being reported. Warr (1987) found that women experience similar levels of physical and psychological ill-health following unemployment. Levels of depression and anxiety are also higher among wives of the unemployed (Cochrane and Stopes Roe 1981).

Going to work, though, may present women who are married and have children with a 'constant juggling act' (Smith 1987). Despite the fact that more women work, the majority of domestic work and childcare still falls on women (*Social Trends* 1990). Cleary and Mechanic (1983) report increased evidence of physical and psychological symptoms in women trying to combine home and work responsibilities. Aneschensel, Frerichs and Clark (1981) found higher rates of depression among women who were employed with young children, and also among single parents. Women too are more likely, especially with the move to community care, to be acting as unpaid carers for other dependent relatives (Equal Opportunities Commission 1982), often resulting in financial difficulties, physical and emotional strain and relationship difficulties (Brody et al 1983).

As more women go out to work they are increasingly exposed to stresses faced mainly by men in the past, such as excessive workload, competitiveness and career structures (Davidson and Cooper 1981). Women are also over-represented in low-status occupations where pay and conditions may be worse and they have little power. This may be aggravated by discrimination and disadvantage (Spencer and Podmore 1987) and sexual harassment (Crull 1982). Poverty has been linked with a higher incidence of mental health problems (Russo 1990). In a study of low-income women with children, insufficient money was found to be a key source of stress (Belle 1982), and this may represent a major problem for single parents.

Rising levels of alcoholism in women have been linked to employment. Seven in every 100 women are now drinking more than 35 units of alcohol weekly, which is defined by the Royal College of General Practitioners as 'harmful drinking'. The highest number of heavy drinkers is in the 17–29 years group, many of whom are from professional, managerial and non-manual occupations, and may be drinking in response to stress or social pressures (Wallace, Brennan and Haines 1987). Of those women receiving treatment, however, a significant number are older housewives (Corrigan 1987). Reasons given for drinking are isolation, feelings of non-achievement and lack of support (Shaw 1980).

It may be that a greater incidence of stressful life events could be responsible for women's greater susceptibility to mental breakdown. Walker (1990) points out the many potential losses that women experience, such as miscarriage, abortion, infertility, childbirth, children going to school, moving with a husband due to work, lost opportunities due to gender. They also take more responsibility for breakdown in relationships and may experience disappointment about the romantic myth of marriage.

Women are also significantly more likely to suffer physical and sexual abuse in our society, which have been linked with a greater risk of mental health problems (Burnam et al 1988). Benward and Denser-Gerber (1975) suggest that up to 40 per cent of female clients in psychiatric hospitals have been sexually abused. Childhood abuse may also lead to later sexual problems. Of a sample of women with sexual problems, 59 per cent were victims of sexual abuse compared with 17 per cent in a control group (Becker et al 1986).

In many cases the abuse may have remained hidden for several years due to the child's fears of punishment, rejection or destroying the family. Urbancic (1987) suggests that the combination of guilt, imposed secrecy and often betrayal by a trusted person means that severe psychological consequences may ensue.

Most people with emotional problems approach their GP for help, and only a minority will receive treatment other than drugs (Goldberg and Huxley 1980). In Miles' sample of 85 people diagnosed as neurotic, only three were not prescribed psychotropic drugs (Miles 1988). In addition, studies have revealed that doctors often feel bored and frustrated by the seemingly vague and trivial complaints brought by female patients (Cooperstock 1976, Stimson 1976). Many feminists are highly critical of the medicalising of what are, in effect, social, emotional and family difficulties: labelling them as psychiatric symptoms and viewing them as individual problems hides the social nature of women's problems (Pollock and West 1984, Miles 1988). Admission to hospital and treatment with medication may represent the 'beginning of a downhill slide' by removing responsibility from the woman (Johnstone 1993). It has also been suggested that much traditional psychiatric treatment attempts to 'readjust' women to stereotypical roles (Barrett and Roberts 1978).

Feminist therapy is seen as an alternative way of helping women with emotional problems. Gender is seen as central to an understanding of mental health problems. However, Ussher (1991) is critical of the view that women's mental illness can be explained solely in terms of male domination, arguing that it is too simplistic, and also that many of the solutions offered are little more than idealistic rhetoric which excludes many women. Nevertheless, she acknowledges that important lessons can be learned from feminist therapy in that it seeks to address social processes rather than just focusing on individual problems. In addition, in contrast to mainstream psychiatry, feminist therapy aims to de-mystify psychological distress and foster active participation and empowerment.

Implications for Nursing

While therapy and counselling often deal with individuals, it is important to recognise the influence of political, social and economic issues on mental health. Nurses should beware of stereotyping patients according to gender or encouraging conformity to traditional roles. Indeed, Savage (1987) suggests that where nurses recognise that gender role expectations are contributing towards ill-health or poor recovery, part of their nursing care must include the provision of information and support to help patients challenge these expectations. Nursing care should also be aimed at working with people to help them to deal with stressful life events and ongoing difficulties.

Despite the high incidence of female psychiatric patients who have been sexually abused in the past, this is an area to which traditional mental health care pays scant attention. Herman (1981) suggests that professionals are often uncomfortable and inept at identifying sexual abuse. Staff should provide a sensitive, caring and confidential atmosphere to enable disclosure and the working through of painful issues if the woman wishes.

Groups may be helpful in work with survivors of abuse (Burgess 1984), and nurses may be in a position to facilitate such groups in psychiatric settings (Urbancic 1989). Urbancic asserts that group work can be therapeutic in the following ways: sharing in an accepting atmosphere; reducing feelings of guilt and deviance; providing an opportunity for learning from peers; offering hope since women are at different stages in coming to terms with their abuse; and developing trust, cohesiveness and positive feelings for other women. Harlett and Scott (1987) describe their experiences of running a group for survivors of abuse in the UK, and stress the need for supervision and support for group leaders. Nurses may also be involved in work with people who have committed sexual offences. Adequate training and supervision is necessary for this demanding and emotive area of work. Details of work with sex offenders can be found in Bancroft (1989).

It can be argued that mental health workers have a responsibility beyond individual care, for broader social action to alleviate factors impeding mental health, both at an individual level and as professionals, for example by lobbying for better childcare and fighting discrimination. The impact of politics and gender needs also to be considered in plans for service development. Faugier (1992), for example, warns against the underlying sexism in allocating funds for 'serious mental illness' rather than the 'worried well' (a label often used to describe sufferers of neurotic illness – usually women). Making such changes will involve mental health workers in examining their own attitudes to male and female roles, and greater attention to gender issues as an integral part of training.

The Relationship Between Mental Health and Sexual Function

A person's sexuality and their mental health are intimately connected, and disruption of one may have serious repercussions on the other. Sexual problems themselves, whether primary or secondary to illness, disfigurement, drugs, childbirth or surgery may result in great unhappiness and anxiety, possibly severe enough to warrant psychological help. Similarly, emotional distress or indeed many psychotropic drugs (prescribed and non-prescribed) may have a negative effect on sexual function. Bancroft (1989) suggests that psychological factors provide the commonest and most important disruption to sexual relations. The incidence of sexual problems among psychiatric patients appears to be high (Crisp 1979, Swan and Wilson 1979, Watson 1979), although sexuality is an area of patients' needs that nurses often ignore.

Sexual dysfunction is generally seen as a disruption to the physical aspects of sex, for example problems of libido, impotence, vaginismus, delayed ejaculation or anorgasmia, but this view reflects 'a narrow understanding of normal sexual function' (Savage 1987). While these aspects of sexuality are important, sexual dysfunction should be seen in a broader sense, including problems in relating to and being emotionally intimate with other people, and feelings about oneself as a sexual being.

The Impact of Depression on Sexuality

The experience of depression is used to illustrate the pervasive influence of emotional distress on sexual health. A more thorough review of the impact of mental health problems and psychotropic medication on sexual function is provided by Bancroft (1989). Feelings of depression may have a devastating effect on sexuality. Beck (1967) found that 61 per cent of his depressed subjects reported loss of sexual interest, compared to 27 per cent of a non-depressed control group. Schreiner-Engel and Schiari (1986) also noted a loss of sexual desire associated with depression, and they question whether this may be due to negative thought processes or to biochemical change. Depression frequently causes a person to feel extremely negatively about themselves, perhaps even to the extent of having delusional ideas about their worthlessness. Sanders et al (1983) found that women's ratings of their sexuality were strongly influenced by general feelings of well-being.

A negative self-concept may lead a person to neglect their hygiene and appearance. They often withdraw into themselves, and consequently significant others may feel less inclined to spend time with them, thus lowering their self-esteem even further. Being labelled as a psychiatric patient can in itself be shattering to an individual's self-esteem (Lemert 1951). Being in hospital, too, may interfere with performance of roles such as parent and breadwinner, further lowering self-esteem and putting a strain on relationships.

Psychotropic drugs used in the treatment of depression may have a negative effect upon sexual performance, possibly exacerbating feelings of inadequacy and anxiety. Mono-amine oxidase inhibitors, used in the treatment of depression, have been associated with ejaculation failure and difficulty in achieving orgasm (Segraves 1985). Tricyclic antidepressants may have a similar effect. In a controlled trial of 36 men and 47 women, Harrison et al (1985) found that 80 per cent of men on phenelzine and 50 per cent on imipramine reported reduced sexual function, compared with 8 per cent who were given a placebo. Fifty-seven per cent of women on phenelzine and 27 per cent on imipramine reported problems, compared with 16 per cent who had a placebo.

Enabling Patients to Meet Sexual Needs

Attention to the sexuality of patients (in its broadest sense), therefore, is an important aspect of holistic care. Miller (1984) suggests that nurses are in a unique position to assess patients' sexual needs and difficulties due to their close relationship with patients and their families. The skills of nurses will be appropriate in most cases rather than specialist services, since the latter tend to use quite a narrow definition of sexuality, often focusing on physical aspects of sex (Savage 1987), and patient problems will commonly relate to more general aspects of sexuality. Baguley and Brooker (1990) see a potential role for CPNs in discussing sexual relations with clients, although it is recognised that some nurses may feel uneasy about broaching sex in the patient's home and indeed the patient may find it intrusive.

Barker (1990) discusses the benefits of assertiveness training for people with long-term mental health problems, which can help them in the development and maintenance of relationships, for example requesting and refusing things, expressing needs and expressing positive and intimate feelings.

Sexual aspects of care should be included in training programmes for nurses, as should the opportunity for students to explore their own sexuality and values relating to sex. Smith-Santopeitro (1980) describes the benefits of a self-instructional module on sexuality in increasing students' knowledge and confidence. If nurses are to become involved in this intimate area of work, they need adequate support and guidance (Chadderton 1988).

In a minority of cases, specialist referral for help with sexual difficulties may be necessary. Nurses rarely take an active role in formal sex therapy but they should be sufficiently skilled to know when referral is necessary, and have an idea of what treatment may involve.

Sex therapy has undergone many changes in the past 100 years. A broad spectrum of approaches is used today, including simple counselling, behavioural methods and psychotherapy, and the past 25 years has seen more work with couples and on relationships generally (Bancroft 1989). More details on approaches to helping people with sexual difficulties can be found in Bancroft (1989).

Issues Relating to the Psychiatric System and Sexuality

Psychiatry as a Controller of 'Deviant' Sexuality

Throughout its history, psychiatry has been closely associated with the regulation of sexual behaviour identified as 'deviant'. Sexual deviance may be defined as sexual behaviour that is 'abnormal, harmful or morally wrong, according to Western culture and fashion' (Gomez 1991). Important in this definition is the notion that ideas about 'normal' sexual behaviour change over time. Ussher (1991) refers to the 'psychiatrising' of sex in the nineteenth century, with people being admitted to hospital for masturbation, pregnancy out of wedlock, homosexuality, frigidity and promiscuity. The influence of Freud, who saw sexuality as a major determinant of behaviour, was important at the time.

Homosexuality provides a good example of how ideas about deviance change over time since, although it still carries some stigma today, it is no longer regarded as a mental illness. There has been some suggestion that mental health problems may be greater among homosexuals (Bancroft 1989), but the impact of stigma and discrimination may well be a highly significant factor. Whereas in the past treatment may have focused on re-orientating the person to heterosexual sex, Bancroft considers that more benefit may be gained by helping people to strengthen the positive aspects of their own sexuality.

Currently, people may receive help in the psychiatric system for a range of behaviours generally regarded as 'deviant', e.g. paedophilia, rape, exhibitionism, frotteurism, voyeurism, fetishism, sado-masochism, transvestitism and transsexualism. However, psychiatric treatment is only appropriate where the person's sexual orientation presents a danger to themselves or other people or is a source of distress to the individual, rather than as a means of ensuring conformity to social norms. Shortage of space prevents a detailed discussion of approaches to helping such individuals, but these are well covered in Bancroft (1989). Buchya (1988) also describes nurses' involvement in behaviour therapy for sexual deviance.

Mental health workers should beware of assuming that all patients are heterosexual, and also need to be aware of the stress caused by discrimination against sexual minority groups. Platzer (1990) suggests that standards of care for gay and lesbian patients are often poor due to lack of knowledge and prejudice among nurses. Exploration of attitudes and prejudices is important in training. Young (1988) discusses the benefits of educational programmes in promoting more positive attitudes to the care of male homosexuals with AIDS.

Psychiatry as the Keeper of Patients' Morality

There is a history in psychiatry of attempts to repress the sexual expression of patients. Ussher (1991) refers to the barbaric practice in the nineteenth and early twentieth centuries of compulsory sterilisation of thousands of mentally ill people to prevent their reproduction. Thomas (1989) suggests that even today, nurses tend either to ignore or deny patients' sexuality, or to impose restrictions on it when it presents problems to the smooth running of the institution.

Lack of privacy and restrictive attitudes of staff tend to mitigate against expression of sexual needs in institutions. This is especially an issue where patients are in hospital for long periods. Thin partitions or curtains and nurses' open access policies give little opportunity for masturbation or for sexual relations with a partner, potentially causing great frustration. Nurses in psychiatry have traditionally occupied a custodial role in relation to patients, monitoring their physical and social activities, as well as acting as the 'keeper of the patient's morality' (Savage 1987). It is important that a balance is struck between protecting those who are vulnerable and ensuring that patients' rights are met. Such issues may necessitate exploration of attitudes and discussion by the team.

Marriage between psychiatric patients has often been met with disapproval due to a belief that they are 'doubling their problems' (Greengross 1976) and to fears of defective genes in children. A retrospective study by Shanks and Atkins (1984) of 22 couples (all ex-psychiatric patients) revealed such fears to be unfounded. The majority rated themselves as happier than before and had spent a significantly shorter period of time in hospital since marriage.

Sexual Harassment in Psychiatric Hospitals

There has recently been considerable concern about reports by patients of sexual harassment and attack in psychiatric units (Feinmann 1988, Cohen 1992, Copperman and Burrowes 1992). Sexual harassment may also be a problem for nurses. It has been suggested that mental health professionals frequently turn a blind eye to this issue (Gorman 1992), and may dismiss patients' complaints, regarding patients as unreliable witnesses.

Mixed wards only came into vogue about 30 years ago, due to a belief that they provided a more realistic reflection of life outside. Questions are now being raised however, about whether mixed wards can really provide a therapeutic environment in which women can recover from mental illness (MIND 1992).

A survey conducted by Thomas (1992) revealed that, while 57 per cent of patients preferred mixed sex wards, 19 per cent would prefer single sex wards, mainly for reasons of safety and privacy. Eleven per cent of women also expressed a preference for female nurses. Thomas recommends the exploration of possibilities for setting up women only wards and areas. Patients should also be able to choose the sex of their key worker.

The MIND campaign 'Stress on Women' calls for an end to sexual abuse and harassment in mental health settings, and for greater attention to be paid to security in hospitals and dealing with sexual abuse. Independent advocacy is seen as one way of ensuring that patients' voices are heard (MIND 1992).

Sexuality and the Patient–Therapist Relationship

Sexuality is often a major factor in the relationship between therapists and patients, yet is largely ignored. In this potentially highly intimate relationship, attraction may develop on either side. Whitley (1978) suggests, however, that when patients make advances to nurses, this may often really be an attempt to validate their sexual identity which has been threatened by illness. Nurses should therefore attempt to encourage expression by patients of their underlying concerns.

Sexual feelings between nurses and patients may interfere with the therapeutic relationship, so it is important that an atmosphere of openness and support is created in order that such feelings can be discussed within the team.

This is especially important in the light of disturbing claims about seduction and sexual assault by therapists of female patients (Masson 1989). Such behaviour is clearly an abuse of patients and a contravention of professional codes of conduct. However, greater recognition of the potential for attraction between patients and staff and more openness may prevent things going so far.

Sexuality and Psychiatric Nursing

There have always been more men in psychiatric than in general nursing. The asylums were traditionally staffed by male attendants, recruited for their strength, in what was predominantly a custodial environment. In 1989, men accounted for almost 30 per cent of the qualified workforce (Department of Health 1991). However, as in nursing generally, a disproportionate number of men occupy the top positions. Stereotyping of men as leaders, failure to value 'female' characteristics in the struggle for professionalism and failure to recognise the needs of women, e.g. for childcare, are all potential contributing factors (Pollock and West 1984).

Part-time staff, who are mainly women, are over-represented in the lower ranks. In 1989, while 33.8 per cent of unqualified staff worked part-time, only 18.3 per cent of qualified psychiatric nurses did so (Department of Health 1991). A survey by Everest, Richards and Hanrahan (1979) of 380 psychiatric nurses trained at the Maudsley Hospital revealed evidence of serious discrimination, in terms of promotion, against those who were not in continuous employment. While 73 per cent of men had 100 per cent continuous careers, only 38 per cent of women did ($P<0.001$). Part-time positions were virtually all at staff nurse or sister level, rather than higher grades. The authors question whether nursing is not still too much geared to the full-time career nurse.

Not only are male psychiatric nurses more likely to occupy top positions, but it seems they are also more likely to attend post-basic courses. Rogers (1983) points out that, while males made up only about 25 per cent of all psychiatric nurses in 1982, they constituted almost 66 per cent of those attending relevant post-basic courses. Brooker and Brown (1986) also found that male nurse therapists exceeded females by $2:1$. It is not clear whether these differences are due to greater numbers of men applying for courses or to bias in admission policies or sponsorship. However, more investigation of this issue is urgently required so that a more appropriate gender distribution is achieved, since the majority of psychiatric patients are women and many express a preference for a female therapist.

Mental Health and Sexuality – a Nursing Care Example

Making use of the literature reviewed, this section uses the example of a woman suffering from depression and gives suggestions to guide nursing care in relation to her sexuality. The full assessment may take some time as trust is gradually established. Nurses need to be aware of making assumptions about another's sexuality, and to show respect and acceptance for the person's moral, personal and religious views. In addition, as McRae and Henderson (1975) stress, 'No one should *have* to discuss sex – nurses need to beware of intrusiveness'. Data can be gathered by talking with and observing the person and how they relate to others, and may involve discussion with their family or significant others. Issues relating to sex and relationships need to be approached with great sensitivity and skill.

Nursing Care of a Woman who is Depressed

Nursing assessment and interventions may focus on gender identity and roles, self-concept and sexual/relationship difficulties. Assessment should extend beyond focusing on individual problems, but should look at the person in the context of her family and society as a whole (Walker 1990).

Questions might include the following:

- Tell me about your life – your work, your home life, marriage/relationships, children.
- How do you feel about your life and your future? Are there any changes you would like to make? Do you feel able to make them?
- What support do you have from other people – your partner, family, friends?
- Tell me about you – how do you feel about yourself as a person? As a woman? As a wife? As a mother? (Explore issues related to confidence, feelings of sexual attractiveness, feeling valued by family/society.)
- Has anything about your depression or being in hospital changed the way you feel about yourself?
- How are things with your partner? Your sex life? Has being ill affected these in any way?
- Are you taking any medication? Has this helped? Have you been aware of any side-effects?
- Tell me about things that have been happening in your life recently (developmental changes, recent life events, ongoing stressors). How do you feel about them?
- Tell me about your past life with your own family. Do you feel that any events from the past have influenced how you feel about yourself now?

In addition the nurse may be able to make use of observations such as how well the client cares for her appearance; how well she relates to others, her partner, her family; how her partner relates to her.

Goals for care
These may include the following:

- Helping the woman to ventilate and to clarify the difficulties/problems she sees with her life at present.
- Helping her to cope better with developmental change, life events and ongoing difficulties.
- Helping her plan and make changes to her life as she sees appropriate.
- Promoting a more positive image of herself.
- Increasing her understanding of the effects of depression and its treatment on herself as a sexual being.
- Helping her family adjust to change.

Nursing Interventions

Nursing care should encompass a broad-based approach in recognition of the multiplicity of factors associated with the onset of depression. Care should be focused not just on the individual but on her as a person in the context of her family and society generally. The approach should be one of 'enabling her to take control of her emotional rescue' (Barker 1990), rather than encouraging passivity and dependence.

The nurse should work in partnership with the woman, enabling her to identify the key factors she sees as presenting barriers to her happiness. She can encourage the woman to consider alternatives and provide support and positive reinforcement as she makes changes in her life. The nurse should beware of stereotyping and of pressurising her into conforming to social roles. Referral to specialists may be necessary to help with practical problems such as housing. Avenues for companionship and support need to be explored, possibly through work with her and her partner, or self-help groups with women in similar circumstances. She may need to work through distressing events from the past, for example sexual abuse, which are interfering with her happiness today. She may wish to make plans for further training, need help seeking employment or wish to get involved in voluntary work.

Fostering a more positive self-image can be done on a simple level by the nurse being available and showing interest and acceptance. She should be encouraged to take a step-by-step approach to recovery, incorporating situations where she can experience success. Positive reinforcement for achievements is helpful, as is encouraging her to recognise her own progress and strengths. When very depressed, she may need encouragement to care for herself, take exercise and mix with others. She may benefit from relaxation or assertiveness training. The nurse should make herself available to discuss sex and relationship difficulties which may be affected by her depression, medication or being in hospital. In some instances, specialist referral for relationship therapy or sex therapy may be helpful. Broader issues to consider in relation to creating a therapeutic environment for such clients are offering a choice of key workers where possible, offering 'women only' space/activities, and having guidelines on sexual harassment for the unit.

Conclusions

Our mental health and sexuality are inextricably intertwined. Aspects of sex and gender are implicated in mental health breakdown, including the influence of sex role stereotypes, gender roles, sexual abuse and sexual dysfunction. Mental health problems themselves can also seriously interfere with our sexuality, whether it be physical acts of sex, self-image and self-esteem, or our ability to form and maintain relationships.

A number of challenges are raised for psychiatric nurses. Patients need to be regarded as sexual beings, and their sexuality needs to be considered in plans for care. A balance needs to be found, though, between recognising patients' rights and protecting those who are vulnerable. We need to address issues of stereotyping and discrimination both in relation to work with patients and in the psychiatric nursing profession itself. The scope of mental health care needs to broaden beyond simply focusing on individual problems to how social factors, including gender issues, may be implicated in breakdown of mental health.

To achieve this, nurses need appropriate education in the form of knowledge and skills, including interpersonal skills. The curriculum should also provide the opportunity for exploration of students' own sexual values. This is an area urgently in need of development in terms of practice, education and research.

References

Aneschensel C, Frerichs R and Clark V (1981) Family roles and sex differences in depression. *Journal of Health and Social Behaviour*, **22**, 379.

Asch S S and Rubin L J (1974) Post-partum reactions. Some unrecognised variations. *American Journal of Psychiatry*, **131**, 870–874.

Baguley I and Brooker C (1990) Schizophrenia and sexual functioning. *Nursing Standard*, **4**, 39, 34–35.

Bancroft J (1989) *Human Sexuality and Its Problems*. Edinburgh: Churchill Livingstone.

Barker P (1990) Breaking the shell. *Nursing Times*, **86**, 46, 36–38.

Barrett M and Roberts H (1978) Doctors and their patients: the social control of women in general practice. In Smart C and Smart B (eds) *Women, Sexuality and Social Control*. London: Routledge and Kegan Paul.

Beck A T (1967) *Depression: Clinical, Experimental and Theoretical Aspects*. London: Staples Press.

Becker J V, Skinner J, Abel G and Cichon J L (1986) Levels of post assault sexual-functioning in rape and incest victims. *Archives of Sexual Behaviour*, **15**, 37–49.

Belle D (1982) *Lives in Stress: Women and Depression*. London: Sage.

Bem S (1974) The measurement of psychological androgyny. *Journal of Clinical Psychology*, **42**, 155–162.

Benward J and Denser-Gerber J (1975) Incest as a causative factor in anti-social behaviour. *Contemporary Drug Problems*, **4**, 325–340.

Bibb J and Chambless D L (1988) Alcohol use and abuse among diagnosed agoraphobics. *Behavioural Research and Therapy*, **24**, 49–68.

Birke L (1986) *Women, Feminism and Biology*. Brighton: Wheatsheaf.

Blaxter M (1987) Self reported health. In Cox B D (ed.) *The Health and Lifestyle Survey*. London: Health Promotion Trust.

Briscoe M (1982) Sex differences in psychological well-being. *Psychological Medicine Monographs*, Suppl. **1**.

Brody E M, Johnsen P T, Fulcomer M C and Lang A M (1983) Women's changing roles and help to elderly patients: attitudes of three generations of women. *Journal of Gerontology*, **38**, 5, 597–607.

Brooker C and Brown M (1986) *A National Follow-Up Survey of Practising Nurse Therapists*. In Brooking J (ed.) *Psychiatric Nursing Research*. Chichester: John Wiley and Sons.

Broverman I, Broverman D, Clarkson F, Rosenkrantz P and Vogel S (1970) Sex role stereotypes and clinical judgements of mental health. *Journal of Consulting Psychology*, **34**, 1–7.

Brown G W and Harris T (1978) *The Social Origins of Depression*. London: Tavistock.

Bruch H (1974) *Eating Disorders: Obesity, Anorexia Nervosa and the Person Within*. London: Staples Press.

Brumberg J (1988) *Fasting Girls: The Emergence of Anorexia Nervosa as a Modern Disease*. Cambridge, MA: Harvard University Press.

Buchya H (1988) Dangerous obsessions. *Nursing Times*, **84**, 35, 59–60.

Burgess A W (1984) Intra-familial sexual abuse. In Humphreys J (ed.) *Nursing Care of Victims of Family Violence*. Reston, VA: Reston Publishing Co.

Burnam M A, Stein J A, Golding J M, Sorenson S B, Forsyth A B and Telles C A (1988) Sexual assault and mental disorders in a community population. *Journal of Consulting and Clinical Psychology*, **56**, 843–850.

Chadderton Z (1988) An investigation to discover nurses' reasons for avoiding an assessment of the activity of daily living, 'expressing sexuality' using the Roper model. London Nursing Studies Project: Polytechnic of the South Bank.

Cleary P D and Mechanic D (1983) Sex differences in psychological distress of married people. *Journal of Health and Social Behaviour*, **24**, 111–112.

Cochrane R and Stopes Roe M (1981) Women, marriage, employment and mental health. *British Journal of Psychiatry*, **139**, 373–381.

Cohen P (1992) High risk mix. *Social Work Today*, **3**, 31.

Cooperstock R (1976) Women and psychotropic drugs. In MacLennan, A (ed.) *Women: Their Use of Alcohol and Other Legal Drugs*. Toronto: Addiction Research Foundation.

Copperman J and Burrowes F (1992) Reducing the risk of assault. *Nursing Times*, **88**, 26, 64–65.

Corrigan E M (1987) Burden D S and Gottlieb N (eds) *Womens' Combined Use of Alcohol and Other Mind Altering Drugs in the Woman Client*. London: Tavistock.

Crisp A H (1979) Sexual psychopathology in the psychiatric clinic. *British Journal of Clinical Practice*, (Suppl.) **4**, 3–11.

Crull P (1982) The stress effects of sexual harassment on the job. *American Journal of Orthopsychiatry*, **52**, 3, 539–544.

Dalton K (1980) *Depression After Childbirth: How to Recognise and Treat Post-natal Depression*. London: Oxford University Press.

Davidson M J and Cooper C L (1981) A model of occupational stress. *Journal of Occupational Medicine*, **23**, 564–574.

Department of Health (1991) *NHS Workforce in England*. London: DOH.

Duker M and Slade R (1988) *Anorexia Nervosa and Bulimia: How to Help*. Milton Keynes, Philadelphia: Open University Press.

Equal Opportunities Commission (1982) *Carers and Services: a Comparison of Men and Women Caring for Dependent Elderly People*. Manchester: EOC.

Everest R, Richards E and Hanrahan M (1979) What happens to Maudsley nurses? A follow up study. *International Journal of Nursing Studies*, **16**, 253–266.

Faugier J (1992) Taking women seriously. *Nursing Times*, **88**, 26, 62–63.

Feinmann J (1988) Corridors of fear. *Nursing Times*, **84**, 39, 16–17.

Fleming O and Seager C P (1978) Incidence of depressive symptoms in users of oral contraceptives. *British Journal of Psychiatry*, **132**, 431–440.

Garai J E (1970) Sex differences in mental health. *Genetic Health Monographs*, 123–142.

Goldberg D and Huxley P (1980) *Mental Illness in the Community*. London: Tavistock.

Gomez J (1991) *Psychological and Psychiatric Problems in Men*. New York and London: Routledge.

Gordon V and Ledray L E (1985) Depression in women. *Journal of Psychosocial Nursing and Mental Health Services*, **23**, 1, 26–35.

Gorman J (1992) *Out of the Shadows. MIND Campaign for Women's Mental Health*. London: MIND publications.

Gove W R and Tudor J F (1972) Adult sex roles and mental illness. *American Journal of Sociology*, **78**, 812–835.

Greengross W (1976) *Entitled to Love*. London: Malaby Press.

Harlett G and Scott C (1987) Breaking the silence. *Nursing Times*, **83**, 37, 59–61.

Harrison W M, Stewart J, Erdhart A A et al (1985) A controlled study of the effects of anti-depressants on sexual function. *Psychopharmacological Bulletin*, **21**, 85–88.

Herman J (1981) *Father–Daughter Incest*. Cambridge, Mass.: Harvard University Press.

Hey V (1985) Getting away with murder: PMT and the press. In Laws S, Hey V and Eagan A (eds) *Seeing Red: the Politics of Pre-menstrual Tension*. London: Hutchinson.

Hibbard J H and Pope C R (1985) Employment status, employment characteristics and women's health. *Women and Health*, **10**, 1, 59.

Home Office (1986) *Criminal Statistics: England and Wales*. London: HMSO.

Huppert F A, Roth M and Gove M (1986) Psychological factors. In Cox B D (ed.) *The Health and Lifestyle Survey*. London: Health Promotion Trust.

Johnstone L (1993) In the same boat. *Nursing Times*, **59**, 27, 30–31.

Kuczynski J H (1980) Nursing and medical students' sexual attitudes and knowledge. *Journal of Obstetric, Gynecological and Neonatal Nursing*, November–December, 339–342.

LaRococco S A and Polit D F (1980) Women and knowledge about the menopause. *Nursing Research*, **29**, 10–13.

Lemert E (1951) *Social Pathology*. New York: McGraw-Hill.

Luggin R, Bensted L, Petersson R and Jacobsen A (1984) Acute psychiatric admission related to the menstrual cycle. *Acta Psychiatria Scandinavica* **69**, 6, 461–465.

Mandell A and Mandell J (1969) Suicide and the menstrual cycle. *Journal of the American Medical Association*, **200**, 792–793.

Masson J M (1989) *Against Therapy*. London: Collins.

McBride A (1988) *Women's Mental Health Research Agenda: Multiple Roles*. Women's Mental Health Occasional Paper Series. Rockville MD: National Institute of Mental Health.

McRae I and Henderson G (1975) Sexuality and irreversible health limitations. *Nursing Clinics of North America*, **10**, 3, 587–597.

Melville J (1984) *The Tranquilliser Trap*. London: Fontana.

Miles A (1988) *Women and Mental Illness*. Brighton: Wheatsheaf.

Miles A (1991) *Women, Health and Medicine*. Milton Keynes: Open University Press.

Miller S (1984) Recognising the sexual health care needs of hospitalised patients. *Canadian Nurse*, **80**, 3, 43–46.

MIND (1992) *Stress on Women. Policy Paper on Women and Mental Health*. London: MIND Publications.

Oakley A (1974) *The Sociology of Housework*. Oxford: Martin Robertson.

Office of Health Economics (1987) *Women's Health Today*. London: OHE.

Orbach S (1976) *Hungerstrike*. London and Boston: Faber and Faber.

Platt S D and Dyer A J (1987) Psychological correlates of unemployment among male parasuicides in Edinburgh. *British Journal of Psychiatry*, **151**, 27–32.

Platzer H (1990) Sexual orientation: improving care. *Nursing Standard*, **4**, 38, 38–39.

Pollock L and West E (1984) On being a woman and a psychiatric nurse. *Senior Nurse*, **1**, 10–13.

Rogers J (1983) *The Career Patterns of Nurses Who Have Completed a JBCNS Course*. London: Joint Board of Clinical Nursing Studies.

Royal College of General Practitioners (1986) *Morbidity Statistics from General Practice 1981–2. 3rd National Survey*. London: HMSO.

Rose S, Lewontin R C and Kamin C J (1984) *Not in our Genes*. London: Pelican.

Russo N F (1990) Forging priorities for women's mental health. *American Psychologist*, **45**, 3, 368–373.

Salokangas R K R (1983) Prognostic implications of the sex of schizophrenic patients. *British Journal of Psychiatry*, **142**, 145–151.

Sanders D, Warner P, Backstrom T and Bancroft J (1983) Sexuality, hormones and the menstrual cycle. In *Changes in Mood and Physical State: Description of Subjects and Method. Psychosomatic Medicine*, **45**, 487–501.

Savage J (1987) *Nurses, Gender and Sexuality*. London: Heinemann.

Schreiner-Engel P and Schiari R C (1986) Lifetime psychopathology in individuals with low sexual desire. *Journal of Nervous and Mental Disease*, **174**, 646–655.

Segraves R T (1985) Psychiatric drugs and orgasm in the human female. *Journal of Obstetrics and Gynaecology*, **4**, 125–128.

Shanks J and Atkins P (1984) Psychiatric patients who marry each other. *Psychological Medicine*, **15**, 372–382.

Sharpe S (1984) *Double Identity*. Harmondsworth: Penguin.

Shaw S (1980) *The Causes of Increasing Drinking Problems Amongst Women: a General Aetiological Survey*. In *Women and Alcohol*. London: Camberwell Council on Alcoholism.

Showalter E (1985) *The Female Malady*. London: Virago.

Smith L (1987) Women and mental health. In Orr J (ed.) *Women's Health in the Community*. Chichester: John Wiley and Sons.

Smith-Santopeitro M C (1980) Effectiveness of a self-instructional module in human sexuality and counselling. *Nursing Research*, **1**, 14–19.

Social Trends (1990) London: Great Britain Central Statistical Office.

Sommer T L (1973) The effect of menstruation on cognitive and perceptual motor behaviour: a review. *Psychosomatic Medicine*, **35**, 515–534.

Spencer A and Podmore D (1987) Women lawyers – marginal members of a male-dominated profession. In Spencer A and Podmore D (eds) *In a Man's World – Essays on Women in Male Dominated Professions*. London: Tavistock.

Stimson G (1976) General practitioners: 'trouble' and types of patient. In Stacey M (ed.) *The Sociology of the NHS. Sociological review monographs no. 22*. Keele: University of Keele.

Swan M and Wilson L J (1979) Sexual and marital problems in a psychiatric outpatient population. *British Journal of Psychiatry*, **135**, 310–314.

Thomas B (1989) Asexual patients. *Nursing Times*, **85**, 33, 49–51.

Thomas B(1992) Involuntary cohabitees. *Nursing Times*, **88**, 49, 58–61.

Urbancic J C (1987) Incest trauma. *Journal of Psychosocial Nursing*, **25**, 7, 33–35.

Urbancic J C (1989) Resolving incest experiences through in-patient group therapy. *Journal of Psychosocial Nursing*, **27**, 9, 5–10.

Ussher J (1991) *Women's Madness: Misogyny or Mental Illness*. Hemel Hempstead: Harvester Wheatsheaf.

Walker M (1990) *Women in Therapy and Counselling*. Milton Keynes: Open University Press.

Wallace P G, Brennan P J and Haines A P (1987) Drinking patterns in general practice patients. *Journal of the Royal College of General Practitioners*, **37**, 30, 354–357.

Warr P (1987) *Unemployment and Mental Health*. Oxford: Clarendon Press.

Watson J P (1979) Sexual behaviour, relationship and mood. *British Journal of Clinical Practice* (Suppl), **4**, 23–26.

Webb C (1992) Sexuality. In Brooking J I, Ritter S A H and Thomas B L (eds) *A Textbook of Psychiatric and Mental Health Nursing*. Edinburgh: Churchill Livingstone.

Whitley M (1978) Seduction and the hospitalised patient. *Journal of Nursing Education*, **17**, 6, 34–39.

Young E W (1988) Nurses' attitudes towards homosexuality: analysis of change in AIDS workshops. *Journal of Continuing Education in Nursing*, **19**, 1, 9–12.

Chapter 8
Asian Women and the Menopause
Vina Mayor

The menopause is a universal experience for women, but their personal experiences are culturally specific and embedded in tradition, folk culture and societal values (Flint 1979, Voda 1982, Wilbush 1988, Morse and Dennerstein 1989, Greer 1991, Golub 1992). In this chapter I will discuss the meanings, myths, symptoms and treatment associated with menopause, and then go on to an account of a project I carried out with a group of Punjabi-Sikh women in the UK. The chapter will conclude with a discussion of the implications of the project for health workers involved with ethnic minority women.

Meanings and Myths of the Menopause

The word menopause is derived from two words: 'mens', meaning monthly, and 'pause', meaning to stop. It refers to the cessation of menstruation and the termination of fertility, two events which may not necessarily happen in tandem. At a pragmatic level, menopause may be defined as the date of the last menstrual period (Brockie 1988, Kelly 1993). The most widely used definition of the menopause is: 'absence of menstrual periods for one year' (Voda 1982). More generally, the term menopause is used to describe the years of transition as ovarian function declines and the body adjusts to changes in hormone levels. The period around the menopause can be divided into three phases: pre-menopause, peri-menopause and post-menopause. Ovarian function begins to decline during the pre-menopause, but there is no change in menstrual function. Changes in menstrual pattern accompanied by vasomotor symptoms are a characteristic feature of the peri-menopause. The post-menopause phase is confirmed when menses have ceased for 12 months.

From a review of the literature (Voda 1982, Bell 1987, Dickson 1990, Golub 1992), the majority of which relates to western culture, it is evident that there

120

is much myth and folklore associated with menopause. For decades, scientific discourses and practices of the western world related to menopause have contributed to the evolution of myths and beliefs which depict a stereotypical picture of menopausal women as deficient, diseased, asexual and having psychological health problems, rather than as women experiencing a naturally occurring event (Bell 1987, Dickson 1990, Gangar and Key 1991, Greer 1991, Kelly 1993). Until recently, menopause was not considered to be an appropriate topic of conversation.

Over the years the medical profession has perpetuated negative attitudes about the menopause (Bell 1987, Greer 1991), viewing women at menopause as passive victims of their changing hormones. Society perceives women in terms of their reproductive system (Greer 1991), as products of its hormones. Most published literature views menopause from a medical perspective which tends to see it as a deficiency disease focusing on dysfunction. However, menopause is not a disease or an illness, but a natural physiological change which is part of the ageing process (Greer 1991, Golub 1992). It is a change that signals a transition from one phase of life to another, specifically the end of the woman's fertility and the end of menstrual cycles, correlating with failure of ovarian function.

Morse and Dennerstein (1989) and Greer (1991), among others, suggest that in western culture there are two prevailing views of menopause. One view suggests that middle-aged women in a youth-orientated, age-denying society experience loss of identity and inner conflict because the meaning of menopause is associated with loss of femininity and physical attractiveness (Greer 1991); or it may be viewed as death of the 'woman inside the woman' with loss of fertility/mothering role (Greer 1991, Miles 1991). Greer (1991) writes that a woman who has been encouraged all her life to think of her reproductive faculty as her most important contribution will be afflicted deeply by the failure of her ovaries. This is a view which is contrary to the experience of women from other cultures, such as the Zulu.

At the same time as menopause, mid-life brings other changes which are not associated with loss of reproductive ability. For many women menopause coincides with the time when children leave the parental home or the death of their parents or partner. It has been suggested that women mourn the 'empty nest' (Morse and Dennerstein 1989). A second view is that the menopause is a social construct resulting from social learning which shapes women's experiences (Davis 1986, Morse and Dennerstein 1989, Greer 1991).

Biological Aspects

Menopause is the result of age-related changes in ovarian function, which gradually decreases female sex-hormone levels to a lower baseline level where they will remain stable for the rest of a woman's life. From about the age of

40 (Bromwich 1989) the ovaries gradually lose their ability to release a follicle. At first, ovulation may stop but menstrual periods may continue until oestrogen production is too low to maintain a menstrual cycle (Kelly 1993).

Menstrual changes, such as the length of the menstrual cycle and the bleeding patterns, vary from woman to woman. There is no predictable pattern, some experience shorter cycles, others have longer cycles, yet others do not experience any change in their cycle length but find that their flow pattern has changed. The irregular patterns of the cycle reflect ageing changes in the ovaries, specifically: reduction in size of ovaries and the concomitant decline in blood oestrogen levels. These changes are gradual, with no clear beginning or end. Ovaries do not cease to produce hormones altogether and they are not the only source of oestrogen. Cells in the central area of the ovary produce androgens, androstenedione and testosterone. Fat cells in the body take up and convert the androstenedione into oestrone (a weak oestrogen) which is further converted by the liver into oestradiol. Both oestrone and oestradiol are positively correlated with weight in post-menopausal women; thus women with more fat make more oestrogen. In addition, the adrenal glands produce a variety of sex hormones.

Menopause occurs in women between 41 and 59 years of age, with the most common age being 50 in industrialised societies (Asso 1983, Fairlie, Nelson and Popplestone 1987, Stott 1991, Golub 1992, Kelly 1993). Contrary to popular belief, there is no relationship between age at menarche and age at menopause (Stott 1991, Golub 1992). Although age of menarche has declined steadily, the mean age at menopause has not changed. Several factors seem to affect age at which menopause occurs: smoking, alcohol consumption and weight may play a role in menopause. Data from two large, independent studies (Ojeda 1989) have confirmed that smokers, as a group, experience earlier menopause. Taller women, women of heavier weight, and women who are currently married (as opposed to those who are widowed, divorced or unmarried) tend to have a later menopause, as do women who have never been pregnant. Conversely, having twins or working outside the home appears to be related to an earlier menopause. The role of lifelong nutrition, stress, illness, race and familial patterns in menopause are not yet precisely understood (Golub 1992), although there is some evidence to suggest that menopause occurs at a similar age in mothers and daughters and in sisters (Bromwich 1989).

Socio-cultural Aspects

Menopausal experiences are influenced by physiological changes, as well as being shaped by social changes going on in a woman's middle-life (Davis 1986). Women differ in the way in which they respond to these changes. Attitudes towards menopause appear to be related to a number of factors, e.g. age, physical health, emotional health and the woman's own menopausal stage. Theisan et al (1991, in Golub 1992) have replicated earlier findings that younger women have more negative attitudes toward menopause than women who were experiencing menstrual changes or were post-menopausal. This may be related to differences in perceptions of women for whom menopause is a hypothetical phenomenon and what is the experiential reality for menopausal women.

Studies (Ojeda 1989, Tlou 1990, Wilbush 1988, Flint 1979) of other societies show that the stereotype of the irrational menopausal woman is not universal, and that western negative reactions to the naturally occurring physiological process of menopause are culturally engendered (Ojeda 1989). For example, South African, Asian and Arabian women welcome the end of childbearing years and have positive attitudes about the menopause.

Datan et al's (1981) study of five Israeli subcultures explored the interplay between culture and women's responses to menopause and middle-age. The study confirmed that women's responses to menopause and middle-age were shaped by the cultures in which they grew up. Datan et al concluded that successful adaptation to menopause seems to require a fit between what the women expect their lives to be like and their actual lives.

Among the Yoruba of Nigeria, passage through menopause enables women to engage in trade and travel. Societies that ascribe a dangerous sexuality to women impose restrictions on women's movements. Menopause rescinds this dangerous sexuality, restrictions on movement (of menopausal women only) lessen (Golub 1992), and women who are traditionally confined in purdah are permitted to travel to distant places on pilgrimage. In eastern cultures, such as India, Japan and China, older women are respected, have a position of authority over the younger generation and are given considerable political and domestic power. In these societies, the work of the daughter-in-law reduces the work of the older woman.

Flint's (1979) study of affluent Rajput women (in mid-India) suggests that they experienced few symptoms other than those confined to the changes in the menstrual cycle, and they positively anticipated menopause. Flint attributes this relative lack of symptoms to the positive changes that menopause brought to their social lives. Menopausal Rajput women are released from purdah, permitted unconditional freedom to socialise in mixed company and achieve status (wisdom, experience, seniority, authority). Flint concluded that, in cultures which sanction role changes that increase a woman's status or decrease her burden, the women do not experience psychological or adverse physiological symptoms with menopause.

In contrast with the 'empty nest syndrome' referred to earlier, Wilbush (1982) reports that menopausal Zulu women substitute 'social' children for biological ones through 'surrogate wombs'. In addition, Zulu women enjoy freedom from contamination by menstrual blood, liberation from being incarcerated and separated in menstrual huts, and assume powerful roles as advisers to the younger wives in the household.

In the Punjabi-Sikh extended family, women in middle-life exercise their growing authority and seniority in choosing the bride/groom for their sons/daughters. With the birth of grandchildren, the Punjabi-Sikh grandmother is more likely to take on the long-term nurturing of grandchildren. Similarly, a study of Botswana women (Tlou 1990) indicates that they perceive menopause as a natural occurrence, a relief from menstrual bother and experiences, and freedom from unplanned pregnancy.

Symptomatology

A wide variety of symptoms are associated with menopause including menopausal hot flushes (MHFs), sweating, headaches, fatigue, vertigo, aches and pains, formication, tingling sensations, insomnia, irritability, weight gain, palpitations, nervousness and depression. MHFs are the most widely cited symptom (Levine-Silverman 1989, Stott 1991, Golub 1992, Mendham and Rees 1992, Kelly 1993) and certain symptoms, such as MHFs, night sweats, insomnia and headaches cluster together. It is possible that these vascular symptoms are related, and that the fatigue and irritability experienced are concomitants of sleep disturbance. Although vasomotor and atrophic symptoms are widely recognised as being characteristic symptoms of menopause correlating with endocrine changes, there is considerable controversy surrounding the plethora of other symptoms (Morse and Dennerstein 1989).

Vasomotor Symptoms

Menopausal hot flushes (MHFs) do not appear to be influenced by the type of menopause, i.e. surgically induced (following hysterectomy) or naturally occurring. Occurrence of MHFs is usually associated with the peri-menopause (Levine-Silverman 1989), although some women report the occurrence of MHFs prior to changes in the menstrual pattern. Voda (1982) noted a positive correlation between perceived duration and reported intensity of MHFs, that is, the longer the duration, the more intense the experience.

Menopausal hot flushes are a sudden sensation of intense heat, occasionally followed by an observable change in skin colour (flushing) and accompanied by profuse sweating. Night sweats are the nocturnal version of MHFs. MHFs usually involve the head, neck and upper body and are sometimes accompanied by other vasomotor symptoms such as palpitations and chills. Some women perceive MHFs as a whole body sensation or affecting different body sites (Voda 1982). Both the frequency and duration of MHFs are extremely variable: some women never have a MHF while others experience them over a period of five to 10 years (Ojeda 1989, Voda 1982, Levine-Silverman 1989, Golub 1992).

Currently, the debate about common triggers to MHFs is inconclusive, as earlier studies (Voda 1982) indicated that none had been identified, whereas Gannon (1988, in Golub 1992) found a significant correlation between MHFs and frequency of daily stresses. Spicy foods, coffee, tea and alcohol have also been identified as common triggers for MHFs (Golub 1992).

Studies investigating the aetiology of menopausal hot flushes (MHFs) have focused on explicating which hormones are the particular triggers involved in MHFs. MHFs and night sweats are both caused by a physiological process involving vasodilatation of cutaneous capillaries. Vasodilatation can lead to a drop in central blood pressure, giving rise to dizzy spells (Gangar and Key 1991). Palpitations are another example of vasomotor instability. The cerebro-vascular arterial tree is sensitive to oestrogens, and the phenomenon of menstrual migraine is well documented (Magos et al 1983, in Gangar and Key 1991). Similarly, some women develop severe migraine-like headaches around the time of the menopause.

Musculo-skeletal Symptoms

At menopause, diminishing oestrogen levels also affect the oestrogen receptors within the musculo-skeletal system (oestrogen receptors have been found in sebaceous glands and hair follicles), resulting in loss of collagen which in turn contributes to dry, thin skin, wrinkles, a progressive decrease in the density of scalp and body hair follicles, brittle nails and breast tissue losing some of its fullness. Menopausal women complain of dry, flaky, itchy skin (formication) which is easily bruised. Diminishing oestrogen levels cause atrophy of the urethral epithelium which may lead to urgency, frequency of micturition, stress continence (Kelly 1993) and atrophic trigonitis (McKay Hart 1991). Other menopausal symptoms, e.g. aches and pains in the joints, joint stiffness or carpal tunnel syndrome, do not appear to have a satisfactory explanation (Gangar and Key 1991, Greer 1991 and Golub 1992).

Osteoporosis is a more sinister but common problem for post-menopausal women. Recent literature (Scane, Sutcliffe and Francis 1991, Golub 1992, Kelly 1993) suggests that up to 50 per cent of (post menopausal) women may be 'silent sufferers' of osteoporosis, meaning that the women may not be aware that their bone mass is adversely affected. Howie (1987) estimated that one in 10 orthopaedic beds in NHS hospitals is taken up by fractures related to osteoporosis.

Osteoporosis, the aetiology of which appears to be declining oestrogen levels, is less common in black women and women with larger bones, but is more common in small-boned, fair skinned women. Several factors have been found to be associated with low bone mass at the time of menopause. Those especially relevant to Asian women are: early menopause (particularly surgically induced), light frame, their race and nutrition. Greer (1991) suggests that osteoporosis is a disease of affluence as well as having a genetic component. She draws her evidence from comparisons of life-styles of western women with those in the Indian sub-continent. Peasant women in the Indian sub-continent have poorer and harsher life-styles, reflecting their poorer socio-economic status, but the impact of regular weight-bearing exercise from walking long distances promotes healthy bone structure. In contrast, women in the west consume a diet rich in red meat (calcium excretion is accelerated by increased protein and phosphorus intake), lead sedentary life-styles, are prone to being overweight and have less weight-bearing exercise, factors which contribute to their predisposition to osteoporosis. Greer's observation supports other literature which indicates that the risks of developing osteo-porosis can be reduced by maintaining adequate exercise and nutrition, as regular exercise promotes muscle tone and bone mass (Ojeda 1989, Scane et al 1991, Golub 1992). Diet is crucial in the prevention of osteoporosis, because if the dietary intake of calcium is inadequate, it is taken from the bones. Adequate dietary intake of calcium can be ensured by consuming foods rich in calcium, especially dairy products.

Psychological Symptoms

Van Keep (1982) suggests that psychological symptoms may be secondary to the primary vasomotor symptoms, e.g. if hot flushes disturb sleep, the client will experience insomnia and fatigue which may result in irritability and nervousness. No difference in depressive symptoms has been found in women of other age groups and women in the menopause (Gangar and Key 1991, Golub 1992) and life stress has more influence than does menopause on both the psychological and somatic symptoms experienced by menopausal women (Asso 1983). However, McKinlay et al (1987) found that depressed women were more likely to report menopausal symptoms such as MHFs, sweats or other problems, and were more likely to seek medical help.

Sexual Symptoms

At menopause, with diminution of oestrogen, vaginal walls become thinner, the vagina loses some of its elasticity, becoming shorter and narrower, and it loses some of its ability to lubricate quickly. In addition, there is a decrease or absence of Bartholin's gland secretion so that the vagina is less moist. When aroused, the pre-menopausal woman takes 6–20 seconds to lubricate, while the menopausal woman takes 1–3 minutes. Should intercourse be attempted before the vagina is adequately lubricated it may be painful and cause bleeding and trauma to the epithelium, with an associated risk of infection. Commercially available water-soluble lubricants such as K-Y jelly can be used as short-term measures to facilitate intercourse, and oestrogen replacement therapy also improves vaginal lubrication. McCoy, Cutler and Davidson (1985 in Golub 1992) report that women approaching menopause who have regular weekly sexual intercourse have higher levels of oestrogen and tend to be free of MHFs or experience milder ones than women who abstain or have more sporadic sexual activity.

Menopause does not mean the end of an active sex life, but a woman's sexuality will be affected if she is experiencing MHFs, dyspareunia and disturbed sleep. If symptoms persist she is less likely to be interested in sex, and her diminution in sexual desire in turn affects her partner's sexuality. Sarrel's (1988 in Golub 1992) study of post-menopausal women reported that 39 per cent of women reported no change in their sexual activity, 14 per cent experienced an increase in sexual activity and 49 per cent reported a decline in sexual activity. Sarrel noted that for some respondents, changes in sexual behaviour were related to a decline in personal interest, while some changes in sexual behaviour appear to be age-related. Age-related decline in sexual activity may also be culture-specific. Tlou (1990) noted that dyspareunia was the least frequently reported symptom in Botswana women, who expect to remain sexually active into senescence.

Therapeutic Responses

Women, universally, are involved in lay healing, either for self care or in caring for others. Lay healing responses are determined by knowledge, level of education and socio-economic status. In addition, self-care responses of women from western and other cultures (Tlou 1990) depend on support menopausal women receive from other women in understanding and validating menopausal experiences.

Simple, practical strategies for coping with MHFs include internal cooling measures such as drinking cool liquids, external measures, involving removing layers of clothes, using an electric fan, opening windows, and psychological measures such as distraction, positive attitude and humour. From a therapeutic perspective, in general, oestrogen or oestrogen-containing compounds have been shown to be the most effective hormonal agent used in the treatment of MHFs to control symptoms and reduce frequency of MHFs (Dennerstein 1989 in Morse and Dennerstein 1989). MHFs can be treated with relaxation and stress-reducing activities (Golub 1992). American studies (Golub 1992) indicate that exercise increases endorphin levels which in turn decrease luteinising hormone secretion from the pituitary, and a concomitant reduction in the incidence and severity of MHFs occurs.

It has been estimated that only 10–35 per cent of menopausal women seek professional help to ameliorate menopausal symptoms (McKinlay et al 1987). The management of physical symptoms, e.g. hot flushes and night sweats, can often alleviate psychological symptoms. Menopausal symptoms may be alleviated by a variety of therapeutic measures such as hormonal or non-hormonal drug therapy. In non-western societies, menopausal symptoms may be managed by using traditional medicines associated with menstrual irregularity (Tlou 1990).

Somatic symptoms of menopause, such as vasomotor symptoms (MHFs and night sweats) and atrophic vaginitis, clearly respond to oestrogen therapy (Good 1989, Scane et al 1991, Golub, 1992, Kelly 1993). Secondary symptoms, such as insomnia, thin skin or vaginal dryness, are also improved by oestrogen therapy. Oestrogen replacement therapy (ORT) carries with it an increased risk of endometrial cancer (Siddle 1986, Scane et al 1991, Golub 1992), but these risks have been countered by the combined use of progesterone (Kiel 1989, Golub 1992).

Unlike the American experience, in the UK the medical profession still remains cautious in its use of hormone replacement therapy (Siddle 1986, Scane et al 1991). Hormone replacement therapy is not a panacea to alleviate menopausal symptoms in their entirety (McKinlay et al 1987). Greer (1991) and Ojeda (1989) advocate that women should have access to accurate, research-based information, including the associated iatrogenic potential of therapies promoted, to make informed choices from the range of therapeutic measures available in order to meet their individual needs.

British Punjabi-Sikh Women's Experiences of the Menopause

The following section of this chapter illuminates the menopausal experiences of six British Asian (Punjabi-Sikh) women. Mindful of the usual ethical considerations, pseudonyms have been used in order to maintain anonymity and confidentiality. Also, the location of the project has not been identified except to state here that it was located in East London during 1990.

The embryonic stages of this project were serendipitous. It started with an informal series of questions in relation to the menopause, put to me by a small group of Punjabi-Sikh women at a social gathering. These women knew each other socially and all knew me either as a health professional or as 'X's daughter'. The latter, within the context of the Indian community, equates with 'being their daughter too'. Thus, they were aware that I was bilingual and spoke both English and Punjabi fluently. What was surprising was that these women approached me in a very public place to talk about menopausal symptoms they were experiencing, as this is an issue which, in my experience, they would not normally discuss with outsiders or in a public place. It appeared that they had decided to approach me primarily because I was 'X's daughter'.

From those earlier conversations it was apparent that not only were the women seeking factual information on the menopause, they were also seeking validation of their experiences (Davis 1986, Tlou 1990). Their requests were couched as follows:

we want to talk about intimate things, things only another woman understands . . .
this kind of talk you do not have with your husband, your daughter or daughter-in-law . . . for months we were hoping to see you around to ask but you never came . . .
. . . we want to know of these things which you (as a female) can tell us from your knowledge (professional knowledge) of these things . . .
for us to understand the talking has to be in Punjabi . . .

Profile of the Group Participants

The group was homogeneous in terms of country of origin, i.e. Punjab in North India; religion (Sikh); living in extended families and marital status (all were married). None had received a formal education but all were fluent and literate in their mother tongue. Between them they had 29 children (range 2–10), and the average age of the women was 51 years. Four were in paid employment, either outside the home or within the home (as machinists). The other two were surrogate mothers for their grandchildren while the daughters-in-law worked outside the home.

Table 8.1 provides a brief profile of the women's menopausal history and Table 8.2 outlines the focus and content of each session.

Session 1

The intention of this meeting was for me to get to know the women and to get a feel of the issues that concerned them. It was important for the women to identify their own health needs and concerns, and to participate actively in identifying an agenda for future meetings. Attempts to set ground rules with the group were futile as the women did not see any gains from the ground rules, and so this was abandoned. The frequency, venue and timing of the meetings were negotiated.

At first, the women did not appear to appreciate or see the need for a series of meetings. Their priority was to obtain factual information on the menopause and they perceived one session of 'questions and answers' as sufficient for that purpose. As the discussion progressed, it became evident that each woman wished to validate her own personal experience by discussing symptoms, e.g. headaches, palpitations, hot flushes, night sweats, joint pains, indigestion or itching; as well as wanting to learn from the experience of others. They recognised that the issues could not be addressed in a single meeting but would require meetings to provide a forum for discussion and debate.

Flexibility and ongoing negotiation permitted a needs-orientated approach. Each session lasted 2–2.5 hours. The first part (lasting approximately one hour) of each session was focused on the topic selected (at the previous meeting), but the second half of the session was more open. Much of the discussion emanated from the focused discussion of the day or from issues discussed at previous sessions.

Session 2

The women had come to the UK in their childbearing years. In the ensuing two to three decades they had acquired a wealth of experience, knowledge

Table 8.1 Profile of the women's menopausal history

Name	Age	Menopausal history
Sukh	56	Had menopause at age 53. Did not report or recall hot flushes, night sweats or any other symptoms
Meeto	56	Had a surgically induced menopause following hysterectomy (for fibroids) at age 52. Has the occasional hot flush (less than one a month). Reports a one-year history of joint pain affecting knees, hips and shoulders. Not on any medication
Amaro	51	Last menstrual period was 3 months ago. Reports vasomotor symptoms of hot flushes and night sweats, the onset of which she attributes to an unexplained weight loss, 13 months ago. Also has mild acne on forehead
Manjit	49	Regular menstrual cycle of 4–5 weeks with occasional flooding. Has always felt fatigued and suffered from headaches at the time of menstruation
Satto	48	Menstrual cycle has been irregular for the last year. Periods are lighter. Reports vasomotor symptoms of hot flushes, palpitations and dizziness
Gurdip	46	No change in menstrual cycle. Has an IUCD in situ

Table 8.2 Focus and content of sessions

Session 1

Focus
Identifying agenda for forthcoming sessions

Content
1. Getting to know the group
2. Ascertaining individual needs
3. Appointing future meetings, confirming venue, etc.

Session 2

Focus
(i) Women's experience of menopause
(ii) Video on gynaecological examination

Content
1. Menopause: women's experiences and perceptions (values clarification)
2. Definition, symptoms, explanatory models
3. Brook Advisory Centre video on gynaecological examination

Session 3

Focus
Expressing sexuality

Content
1. Self- and body-image in middle-age years
2. Sexual health: e.g. managing atrophic vaginitis and urethral syndrome
3. Myths and realities of contraception

Session 4

Focus
Women's health issues

Content
1. Screening: e.g. mammography, self breast examination, cervical cytology
2. Healthy eating: prevention of osteoporosis, preventing obesity, cardio-vascular disease and hypertension
3. Exercise: weight-bearing exercise to promote healthy bone formation, prevent osteoporosis and promote cardio-vascular health

Session 5

Focus
Self-help strategies

Content
1. Half-hour exercise routine
2. Self-help, e.g. support group; using alternative therapies, e.g. massage, using evening primrose oils, etc.
3. Identifying health needs as opposed to personal needs
4. Health care provision

Session 6

Focus
Dealing with unfinished business and moving on

Content
1. Half-hour exercise routine (requested by the women)
2. Filling in gaps, revisiting aspects of previous sessions as necessary
3. Role-playing interview with GP/Practice Nurse to enable the women to articulate and rehearse the interaction
4. Evaluating the sessions
5. Leaving the door open

Evaluation
1. Would like to access health education leaflets and videos, especially those available in mother tongue
2. Asked me to produce audio- or video-taped information on the subject (a 15-minute audio-tape has been produced and is being piloted)
3. Feedback from sessions 2, 3 and 4 were very positive in that the women felt the most important and salient issues had been addressed in the mother tongue at a level which they understood. All six stated that they were better informed about the menopause as a result of the sessions
4. Session 5 was evaluated less well primarily because they did not feel that health care services would be responsive to their needs

Note: At each session time was set aside for open group discussion and the topic for the following meeting was agreed upon.

and information about pregnancy and fertility issues. As will be seen from the excerpts, each woman had a certain knowledge of the Punjabi myths associated with menopause.

Menstruation folk-speech (Golub 1992, Davis 1986) exists universally. Punjabi euphemistic expressions illuminating menstruation are: visitor/monthlies/bleeding/unwell/cloths are here, time of month, my turn has come, rest days. Similarly the menopause is referred to in Punjabi folk-speech as 'all those woman's troubles are now finished', 'monthlies have gone', 'now I have started my old woman phase'. Meanings of menopause were articulated by the women in terms of others' experiences, symptoms, changes of life-style and other concepts.

When you get the change, your face becomes spotty, your hair turns white. (Manjit)

The old ones always have headaches, you know women who are a bit soft can go mad. I don't want to go mad. (Satto)

They say that once your monthlies stop, you body is less energetic and softer . . . the skin is soft like cotton wool and marks easily (meaning bruising). (Satto)

Menopause is the time for leisure . . . daughters are married . . . daughters-in-law are in charge of the housework. (Sukh)

I was so pleased to finish with this dreadful business of periods, I thanked God a million times. It gives me freedom. (Sukh)

When I lived in India, I never knew anybody who had the menopause. When I got married, I was nearly 18, my youngest brother was three (referring to her parents' sexuality). I don't know how old my mother or aunts were at their menopause. (Gurdip)

There was a certain vagueness about the meanings and myths of menopause for these women. One reason for this may be that, having migrated to the UK in their childbearing years, as a group these women did not observe their older relatives' experience during menopause. Lack of reference to loss of reproductive ability was unexpected. These women were from a culture which encouraged them to consider their reproductive ability as the most important contribution of their lives (Greer 1991), yet they were very accepting of the functional change of their body from fertility to non-fertility. Further discussion indicated that loss of biological fertility was compensated by grandparenthood.

The women identified the onset of menopause as being between 47 and 58 (a later onset than suggested in literature for women in industrialised societies). They estimated the duration of menopause on the basis of folklore as 6 months to 10 years (most sources suggest it last 2–3 years).

Symptoms associated with the menopause were varied and individual. Vasomotor symptoms, as well as the unpredictability of the menstrual pattern were considered to be of importance:

Have I finished with the monthlies or haven't I, how will I know when I have finished . . . this body is fickle, it does not know how to behave, last monthly was 3 months ago . . . heavy for a day, nothing for 2 days then a smear for 2 more days. (Amaro)

When the face goes red (referring to a hot flush), the family want to know why I am so angry. What do I say? When I first started the sweats, my daughter-in-law wanted me to ring the doctor for treatment. When I spoke to the doctor (GP), she just said all women get these problems, it is your age. (Meeto)

On further questioning it became apparent that consultation with the general practitioner had not added much to her understanding of the menopause. Instead her symptoms were dismissed as part of ageing, reflecting the polarity in medical attitude (Greer 1991, Golub 1992).

Overall, the women did not describe feelings of depressed mood, weepiness or irritability but they had experienced physical discomfort, e.g. headaches, joint pains, backache, leg pains, indigestion, constipation, 'feeling heavy from the navel downwards' (abdominal congestion). None of the women thought the symptoms were important enough to warrant consulting the GP, their rationale being that the symptoms had not interfered in their daily lives in any major way.

Lay Management and Attitudes to Menopause

Management of night sweats and hot flushes generated a rich discussion. On one hand the women feared feeling chilled after hot flushes or night sweats, as sweats are associated with febrile illness for which they would normally take to bed with hot water bottles and extra blankets, on the other they were seeking confirmation of the myth that sweating which accompanied hot flushes was some kind of divine protection from serious ill health:

> . . . the wise woman's saying is that if you get the sweats, you are lucky because then you will not get any other illness. (Manjit)

A number of strategies, which included taking a supply of drinks to the bedroom, having lighter bedding and night wear, having a supply of spare bedding and night wear easily accessible to minimise disturbance, were suggested. Leaving the window open overnight, in the winter, was not acceptable to the women concerned:

> Night sweats are problematic. I don't know how to deal with them. The family think I have gone mad, they never know what time I will start cooking. I get up 2 or 3 times a night to get a drink. When the sweats come, I want to leap out of my skin . . . I want to open the windows wide but we people believe that if our joints get a chill I shall be bed ridden or be paralysed even. (Meeto)

Countless myths associated with hysterectomy circulate within the Indian community. A prevailing view exists that surgically induced menopause ensures a symptom-free passage through menopause:

> There is no medication in the world to stop this mess (menstruation), you have to wait your natural time. Ghorian (Caucasian/indigenous women) are okay, very lucky, they have the 'big operation' (referring to hysterectomy) whenever they feel ready for it. I know because two English women who work with me had the 'big operation'. Operation is no good, makes your body go soft (prone to aches and pains) and you get old quicker. Indian women only get sent to be cleaned up inside (meaning D & C). (Satto)

At first the women found it difficult to believe that surgically induced menopause was not symptom-free. Nevertheless the myth associated with Indian women being referred for dilatation and curettage (D & C) of the uterus could not be altered:

> If the monthlies get less (diminished flow), it is better to eat hot foods (foods which Indians regard as having hot properties) not dabhra, more like panjiri (made from butter, semolina and nuts). Hot foods clean the uterus out by increasing the blood flow, because you don't want the old blood which is bad left in, it brings illness (headaches, lethargy, arthritis). (Manjit)

Some women believe that MHFs are caused by 'too much or bad blood' and welcome purifiers in the form of hot foods to strengthen the body and get rid of impurities (Davis 1986). Evidence of lay healing and self-care interventions (Tlou 1990) was minimal, limited to treatment of menopausal acne:

> I treated the face spots (acne) with besan and haldi (gram flour and turmeric) but even more spots have come up. I know I should not eat spicy food, it gives me indigestion and makes my skin erupt in spots, but without spices food is tasteless (sighs) really you don't expect to have these problems at this age . . . don't look smug, your turn will come (this last comment was directed at me). (Amaro)

Although Bransen (1992) contends that lay women perceive and articulate natural life-cycle changes in terms of medical diagnosis, the impact of culture as a variant does not appear to be taken into account. In contrast to Bransen's thesis, these six Punjabi-Sikh women did not medicalise their symptoms, instead perceiving them as a natural part of ageing.

Therapeutic interventions including hormone replacement therapy, complementary therapies and non-hormonal therapy, were discussed but perceived negatively by the person concerned:

> You are just like the ghorian (meaning Caucasian, indigenous women), very keen to go and get the tablets . . . like the ghorae-loke (white people) you don't think that this body should have the occasional ache or pain . . . first sign of problem and you run to the doctor . . . you never stop to think what the tablets will do to your inside . . . western medicine is very hot, not everybody can tolerate it . . . medicines all the time is not good for your body, hormones or pormones (whatever you call them) will make them 100 times worse . . . desi (traditional) medicine is more gentle and natural for your body. (Amaro)

Discussion confirmed that every woman's menopause is different. As far as the women were concerned they were gaining from menopause. They welcomed the associated seniority (white hair correlates with wisdom); status of an elder; privilege, respect and prestige of being consulted as a senior of the community; increased leisure time as daughters-in-law take over the domestic chores; and authority of managing the household.

Session 3

Contrary to Lynam's (1985) experience, the women did not hesitate to discuss matters of a personal, private and intimate domain with a member of the same ethnic community. They were candid in sharing details of experiences, worries and concerns within the context of the menopause. However, when I asked probing questions in order to clarify intimate issues further, the women were initially reluctant, as they perceived my age (late 30s) as a barrier to 'opening up' to me.

Issues raised were atrophic vaginitis, dyspareunia, decreased libido and contraception. Amaro, who was keen to stop using contraception, was most disappointed to discover that conventional advice is to continue for one year after the last menstrual period (LMP) for women over 50 (Kubba 1990). Discussion on this issue was fuelled by the advice Sukh had been given by her GP, who had apparently advised her that she need not use contraception after 6 months:

> When we get together now (meaning sexual intercourse) he does not use rubbers (condoms). Doctor told me it was okay to stop the rubbers as I had not seen the monthly for 6 months. (Sukh)

It would appear that the women had relied on three modes of contraception: barrier method (condoms), IUCD or coitus interruptus. The debate on contraception advanced to include discussion about their sexuality. More personal and intimate disclosures followed. Negative changes in sexual behaviour appear to be related to atrophic vaginitis (McCoy et al 1985 in Golub 1992), decline in personal interest (Sarrel 1988 in Golub 1992) or as secondary symptoms of vasomotor instability:

> Sex is okay, but it leaves a burning feeling inside, no, no there is no bleeding, I don't need the doctor, it will get better, maybe I need a rest from sex, I am embarrassed to see the doctor with this, doctors these days are as young as my children, alright, oh leave it alone, I will see him to get some cream. (Satto) [N.B. She agreed to consult the GP, on condition that I either accompanied her or wrote a note on her behalf.]

Increase in sexual activity (Sarrel 1988 in Golub 1992) was illuminated by the following commentary:

> Stopping monthlies is like getting a bonus pay packet . . . I enjoy sex more now . . . no rubbers (meaning condoms), no coils (referring to IUCD), no pills to burn your insides. Before if he did not use anything, he use to come out quickly (coitus interruptus), which I didn't like but what can you do. (Sukh)

Session 4

A key issue explored in Session 4 was that of cervical cytology. Of the six women, only one had had a cervical smear. The others did not know what cervical cytology was or how they could access the service. Two recent studies of Asian and ethnic women by Doyle (1991) and McAvoy and Raza (1988) have shown that low uptake is associated with lack of knowledge of the existence of the service and lack of understanding and knowledge of the importance of screening. Balarajan and Soni Raleigh (1993) refer to data which indicate that cervical cancer is by far the commonest malignancy in women in the Indian sub-continent. Data such as these are cause for concern and further investigation is needed to determine whether UK Asian women reflect the higher incidence of their country of origin.

Session 5

All six women held low expectations of health professionals, other than GPs. GPs, rather than health visitors, district nurses or practice nurses, were perceived as the primary point of contact. All experienced GPs as gatekeepers to other services. Although the women were registered with GP practices where at least one of the GPs spoke an Asian dialect, e.g., Punjabi, Hindi or Urdu, all had experienced GP consultations via interpreters. While they recognised that their need for interpreter services made it more difficult for them to access health care easily, they were concerned about confidentiality, feeling acutely embarrassed to reveal personal and intimate details via young interpreters. They did not want their private and personal business to be a source of gossip in the community, a finding which confirms Anderson's (1987) Indo-Canadian study. Also they found that protracted interviews were frustrating. All six women were reluctant to use relatives/friends as mediators or advocates on their behalf (Anderson 1987). As their literacy was confined to Punjabi, it was virtually impossible to access high-quality printed literature (in mother tongue) on health issues. Often educational materials which have been translated are of poorer quality both in terms of presentation and the imparted message. At the time of this project (1990), there were no materials available on the menopause in Punjabi.

The women felt that their health was poorer than that of indigenous women. They believed that they were not taken seriously by the GP, the GP did not give them enough time and language barriers affected them adversely, but the sex of the doctor was not perceived as problematic. One of the women had consulted a locum GP for her chronic backache and joint pains and was advised to go to a keep fit class. She viewed the suggestion as being wholly inappropriate and irrelevant to her actual needs. The women used this cameo case study as an exemplar of lack of understanding demonstrated by health professionals to their health needs. They saw GPs as gatekeepers to specialist services but did not see nurses (practice nurse, HV, DN, CPN, etc.) as having a role in health care delivery or health promotion. This may have been partly due to a lack of understanding of the role/s of other health professionals.

Exercise was a low priority for the group until links between osteoporosis and menopause were explored with reference to aetiology, predisposition and preventative measures. The women were receptive to dietary advice to ensure recommended dietary intake of calcium, and willing to increase the level of weight-bearing exercise through daily walks.

Conclusion

The management of the sessions was at times a frustrating experience for me because the women were often late in arriving, and brought infant/toddler grandchildren with them. It appeared that the women had difficulties with their time management because they had not shared the purpose and focus of their meetings with their spouses or other members of the family, highlighting the sensitive nature of issues related to menopause.

It is not feasible to generalise the findings of this small study but, irrespective of the small sample size, the project nevertheless identified important issues which require further consideration and research. Findings indicate that the menopause for Punjabi-Sikh women, like their western counterparts, is shrouded in myths and taboos. In contrast to their western sisters, Punjabi-Sikhs regard menopause as a natural event, occurring concurrently with other mid-life events.

It is imperative that health professionals access culture-specific and relevant data. In order to offer meaningful experiential validation and sensitive, emotional support within the cultural context and language of the menopausal client, health professionals such as health visitors and practice nurses may be required to work alongside mother tongue mediators or acquire skills in community development work in order to cascade health information through the lay network.

Health professionals should empower women to make decisions through sharing knowledge and facilitating access to accurate, research-based information on the menopause, its variability and individuality in order that women may determine whether their own menopause is normal or abnormal (Greer 1991). Decisions about therapeutic interventions should be joint decisions between client and health professional, but led by the client. In addition, women need to know where and from whom this information can be accessed. Women whose mother tongue is not English are at present disadvantaged in their capacity to access health care and health literature. A specialist data base is required to hold and disseminate information on research and education materials in minority mother tongue languages.

Menopausal experiences of ethnic minority women cannot be subsumed under those of western women but need to be examined from the ethnic minority women's viewpoint in order to understand the relationship of culture, ethnicity, class and gender with menopausal health experiences (Douglas

1992). Unless health professionals in the primary health care sector identify menopause as an important issue for ethnic women's health, research-based literature will continue to be lacking. To meet the needs of menopausal women, health professionals need to discern and incorporate research findings into their clinical practice (Levine-Silverman 1989).

Nurses in all settings, particularly those working in the community, need to recognise that if they are to offer holistic and needs-orientated care to ethnic minority clients in relation not only to the menopause but to all aspects of health care, then they need to:

- develop instruments and tools to collect culturally sensitive data;
- adopt a community development approach to initiate health promotion strategies;
- work collaboratively with other agencies to provide culturally sensitive and meaningful health care.

The findings of this project should also be noted by purchasers of health care for incorporation into annual specifications and budgets.

References

Anderson J M (1987) Migration and health: perspectives on immigrant women. *Sociology of Health and Illness*, **9**, 4, 410–438.

Asso D (1983) *The Real Menstrual Cycle*. Chichester: John Wiley and Sons.

Balarajan R and Soni Raleigh V (1993) *Ethnicity and Health: A Guide for the NHS*. London: Department of Health.

Bell S E (1987) Changing ideas: the medicalisation of menopause. *Social Science and Medicine*, **24**, 6, 535–542.

Bransen E (1992) Has menstruation been medicalised? Or will it never happen. *Sociology of Health and Illness*, **14**, 1, 99–112.

Brockie J A (1988) The menopause. *Nursing*, **3**, 25, 955–957.

Bromwich P (1989) *Menopause: Treating the Symptoms*. Wellingborough: Eqution in association with the BMA.

Datan N et al (1981) *A Time to Reap*. Baltimore: Johns Hopkins University Press.

Davis D L (1986) The meaning of menopause in a Newfoundland fishing village. In Morse, J M (ed.) *Qualitative Health Research*. London: Sage Publications.

Dickson G L (1990) A feminist post-structuralist analysis of the knowledge of menopause. *Advanced Nursing Science*, **12**, 3, 15–31.

Douglas J (1992) Black women's health matters: putting black women on the research agenda, Chapter 2. In Roberts H (ed.) *Women's Health Matters*. London: Routledge.

Doyle Y A (1991) A survey of the cervical screening services in a London district including reasons for non-attendance. Ethnic responses and views on the quality of the service. *Social Science and Medicine*, **32**, 953–957.

Fairlie J, Nelson J and Popplestone R (1987) *Menopause: a Time for Positive Change*. London: Javelin Books.

Flint M (1979) Male and female menopause: a cultural put on. In Voda A M et al (eds) 1982 *Changing Perspectives on Menopause*. Austin: University of Texas Press.

Gangar K and Key E (1991) Presentation of menopausal symptoms. *Well Woman Team*, **1**, 4, 8–9.

Golub S (1992) *Periods: From Menarche to Menopause*. London: Sage Publishers.

Good R S (1989) Oestrogen in menopausal mood disorders: a review of the literature and commentary. In Demers L M et al (eds) *Premenstrual, Postpartum and Menopausal Mood Disorders*. Baltimore: Urban and Schuarzenberg.

Greer G (1991) *The Change. Women, Ageing and the Menopause*. London: Hamish Hamilton.

Howie G (1987) Sparing the flushes. *Nursing Times*, **83**, 49, 51–53.

Kelly J (1993) Effects and treatment of the menopause. *British Journal of Nursing*, **2**, 2, 123–125.

Kiel D (1989) Post menopausal oestrogen and hip fractures. *Geriatric Medicine Today*, **8**, 2, 46–56.

Kubba A (1990) Contraception at the menopause. *Well Woman Team*, **1**, 3, 7–9, 12.

Levine-Silverman S (1989) The menopausal hot flash: a Procrustean bed of research. *Journal of Advanced Nursing*, **14**, 939–949.

Lynam M (1985) Social support developed by immigrant women. *Social Science and Medicine*, **21**, 3, 327–333.

McAvoy B R and Raza R (1988) Asian women: contraceptive knowledge: (i) attitudes and usage, (ii) contraceptive services and cervical cytology. *Health Trends*, **20**, 11–17.

McKay Hart D (1991) Hormone replacement therapy and osteoporosis in general practice. *Update Postgraduate Centre Series: Osteoporosis*, 23–26.

McKinlay J B et al (1987) Health status and utilisation: behavior associated with the menopause. *American Journal of Epidemiology*, **125**, 110–127.

McKinlay S M, McKinlay J B and Avis, N E (1989) The Massachusetts Women's Health Study: A longitudinal study of the health of mid-aged women. *Psychology of Women Newsletter*, **16**, 2, 1–3. American Psychological Association.

Mendham C and Rees C (1992) Menopause: a positive change. *Nursing Times*, **88**, 12, 34–35.

Miles A (1991) *Women, Health and Medicine*. Oxford: Oxford University Press.

Morse C and Dennerstein L (1989) Psychological aspects of the climacteric. In Demers, L M et al (eds) *Premenstrual, Postpartum and Menopausal Mood Disorders*. Baltimore: Urban & Schuarzenberg.

Ojeda L (1989) *Menopause Without Medicine*. London: Thorsons (Grafton Books/ Harper Collins Publishers).

Scane A C, Sutcliffe A M and Francis R M (1991) Management of established osteoporosis. *Update Postgraduate Centre Series: Osteoporosis*, 29–32.

Siddle N (1986) Hormone replacement therapy: who should be treated? *Medical Dialogue*, **104**, 11 September.

Stott P (1991) *Teamwork: The Menopause and HRT. Study Book*. Surrey: Medicom (UK) Ltd.

Tlou S D (1990) *The Experiences of the Perimenopause among Botswana Women*. University of Illinois Press.

Van Keep P A (1982) The menopause. In Dennerstein L and Burrows G D (eds), *1983 Handbook of Psychosomatic Obstetrics and Gynaecology*. New York: Elsevier.

Voda A M (1982) Menopausal hot flash. In Voda A M, Denners M and O'Donnell, S E (eds). *Changing Perception on Menopause*. Austin: University of Texas Press.

Wilbush J (1988) Climacteric disorders – historical perspectives. In Studd, J W W and Whitehead, M I (eds) *The Menopause*. Oxford: Blackwell Scientific Publications.

Chapter 9
Gender, Sexuality and Heart Disease
David Shaw

Introduction

There can be little argument that coronary heart disease (CHD) is a major health issue throughout the UK. For example, we know from OPCS figures (OPCS 1993) that myocardial infarction results in almost 83,000 premature deaths every year in Wales and England alone. These figures also tell us that CHD is the major cause of premature death in men and in women, both when taken together and independently, though this varies according to the age group under consideration. The importance of CHD is now fully recognised at all levels and is identified by the government as a key area for action in its recent White Paper, *The Health Of The Nation* (DoH 1992).

Neither can there be much doubt that gender is a major health issue, playing as it does a major part in health and well-being throughout life: the influence of gender on health and the role of the nurse within this have been pointed out by a number of authors (e.g. Webb 1985).

What does seem remarkable, however, is that health workers have been very slow to relate the two issues of gender and CHD. Gender issues within CHD have seldom been raised or even acknowledged, and this blind spot applies to clinical nurses as well as those who conduct research and those who write.

Although issues of gender, sex and sexuality permeate all aspects of CHD, this chapter will focus on one specific aspect: gender issues in the psycho-social impact of heart attack. A central message which will emerge from this chapter is that CHD is seen by professionals and the general public alike as being very much a mans' disease. Gender issues in CHD have been studiously ignored by researchers, practitioners and policy makers. This should be viewed by nurses as a matter of serious concern, since this masculine or 'androgenic' bias threatens to seriously disadvantage women.

140

Women and Coronary Heart Disease

The view of CHD as a man's disease is not consistent with the facts. Although mortality continues to be highest among middle-aged men, it is also extremely high among some groups of women, notably the manual classes (Marmot and McDowell 1986) and the traditional gender gap is narrowing. The modest decrease in mortality which has occurred in the UK since 1978 has been more pronounced in men than in women, and indeed mortality has increased among working-class women during this time (Marmot and McDowell 1986). Furthermore, differences in the natural history of the disease may mean that the prevalence of non-fatal CHD is even more common among women than the mortality rates would suggest: one major study found an equal incidence of angina in men and women (Haynes and Feinleib 1980).

The question of why CHD is more common in certain groups, and why the traditional gender gap is narrowing, is beyond the scope of this discussion; however, suffice it to say our perceptions have not kept pace with the changing reality.

Viewing CHD through a Masculine Prism

It is clear from the literature that the vast bulk of CHD research demonstrates a very consistent bias towards men. This bias extends throughout all areas of CHD research and has seriously distorted our perception of the problem (e.g. White 1985, Bartley, Farrant and Russell 1986, Khaw 1993). For example, in the field of aetiology there is paucity of research involving females despite known and suspected differences in risk factor susceptibility. This masculine bias is coupled with a bias toward biomedical factors and a corresponding neglect of psychological and socio-occupational factors, which may be more important in explaining the prevalence of CHD in both sexes than are conventional biomedical risk factors (Marmot et al 1978, Haynes and Feinleib 1980, Lynch and Oleman, 1981).

As indicated above, the masculine view of CHD is not confined to the research community, but may well also be shared by clinicians. For example, recent studies have shown that physicians frequently treat women differently to men. Women presenting with cardiac symptoms are less likely to be investigated and, even when CHD is demonstrated, they are less likely to undergo coronary artery bypass surgery or angioplasty (e.g. Steingart et al 1991, Petticrew, McKee and Jones 1993).

These studies raise important questions about physicians' perceptions, attributions and beliefs about cardiac symptoms and findings in women, and may well mean that women are being under-investigated and under-treated. It may be that womens' symptoms are not taken as seriously as mens', or that physicians tend to attribute them to non-cardiac causes.

Alternative Ways of Viewing Coronary Heart Disease

Price (1983) attempts to explain the masculine image of CHD by examining its metaphorical character, and argues that the Type A (or Coronary Prone Personality) is a metaphor for masculinity as defined by western society, i.e. aggressive, competitive and multiphasic. She argues that CHD emanates from man's instrumentalism which, as defined by Parsons (1951), is descriptive of the male gender role.

It is certainly true that Type A and the traditional view of masculinity overlap considerably, and it is also the case that Type A characteristics are more common in men than women, though women who work outside the home are likely to have higher Type A scores than other women (Waldron 1978a). Working from the theory that Type A is a behaviour pattern which proves highly functional in the educational and socio-economic domains (e.g. Chesney and Rosenman 1980), Waldron reasons that the increased number of women now pursuing careers outside the home may be resulting in increased Type A behaviour and a corresponding increase in CHD, though she concedes that we must await clear evidence of this happening (Waldron 1978b).

Furthermore, it is evident that Type A behaviour may be dysfunctional in those areas of life which involve affective interpersonal relationships (e.g. Burke, Weir and Duwors 1979). Price (1983) argues that there is a link between CHD and gender roles in which affective interpersonal expression is taboo, i.e. the traditional western masculine role in which emotional expressiveness is actively discouraged (Greenglass 1982). The importance of affective social support in health and illness is well established (House 1981).

The conclusion of this line of argument is that men or women who are highly masculine by traditional western standards are at higher risk of developing CHD than less masculine individuals. It also raises the question of whether masculinity or femininity may be important in influencing the psycho-social recovery of heart attack victims, and this idea will be explored later.

Psycho-social Adjustment Following Heart Attack

This discussion will focus here on psychological and social adaptation following heart attack. There is now an impressive body of knowledge which describes and seeks to explain the psycho-social experience of having a heart attack, the extent to which victims are able to adapt to their changed circumstances, and re-establish their psychological and social equilibrium. This body of knowledge is derived from many hundreds of studies over the past 30 years. However, an examination of this research betrays a tremendous gender bias: very few studies even included women in their samples, let alone attempted a comparison of experiences and psycho-social needs with those of men.

The result of this gender bias is that we know very little about the psycho-social experience of women following heart attack, and are therefore poorly placed to anticipate and meet their needs. In contrast to this, a wealth of data testifies to our understanding of the psycho-social needs of men following heart attack, and intervention studies have shown how much psycho-social morbidity can be avoided. Thus, the fundamental questions which need to be addressed relate to the possibility of male–female differences in the psychological impact of heart attack and the possibility that, if such differences are found to exist, women may have different needs and problems with consequent implications for health professionals. The following account will assess the extent to which previous research may provide answers to these questions.

An extensive literature search revealed only two studies which set out to compare male and female post-coronary patients, and a further study specifically looking at sexual activity in post-coronary women. In addition to this, the voluminous literature on male post-coronary patients included descriptions of a few research projects which have included women in their samples and, in even fewer cases, distinguished between men and women when discussing their results. The following discussion will focus on these fragments of information, on the three studies referred to above, and will attempt to place them within the wider context of the established knowledge base derived from studies on post-coronary men.

Briefly, the research evidence indicates that current practice in the rehabilitation of heart attack victims is generally faithful to the medical model, and despite its success in minimising medical complications and physical symptoms, etc., there exists abundant evidence of widespread psycho-social morbidity which seriously reduces the quality of life in surviving male heart attack victims. This morbidity is normally assessed according to four measurable outcomes: mood state; return to work; family relationships; and the resumption of sexual activity.

Mood State

State anxiety levels in the period immediately following heart attack have been extensively studied in men. Apart from being unpleasant, high levels of anxiety during this stage are known to be associated with poor medical outcome and with long-term psycho-social distress.

Studies have identified that initial anxiety is caused by fear of sudden death and fear of recurring chest pain (Baxter 1975). Anxiety tends to peak on admission to the Coronary Care Unit (CCU), on transfer from the CCU to the ward, and around the time of discharge from hospital (Thompson et al 1987). The high anxiety which exists in the first few days is amenable to nursing interventions as reflected in a range of physiological and psychological measures (Toth 1980) and as reflected in reduced likelihood of medical complications (Klein et al 1968). Studies have also shown that individuals vary in the extent to which they exhibit coping mechanisms such as inappropriate sexual behaviour and denial. For example, studies have shown denial to be effective in reducing anxiety (e.g. Gentry et al 1972) but negatively associated with compliance behaviour (e.g. Croog, Shapiro and Levine 1971), both of which have implications for nurses.

Other studies have examined the medium- and long-term psychological effects of heart attack, and have identified anxiety and depression as being widespread. For example, Lloyd and Cawley (1978) found that 35 per cent of their sample of 100 men suffered 'psychiatric morbidity' one week following their heart attack, and Wynn (1967) found considerable and 'unwarranted emotional distress' in 50 per cent of his sample of 400 men over a period of two years. Studies such as these have identified high-risk groups along with prescriptions for intervention (e.g. Naismith et al 1979). It has been repeatedly demonstrated that these medium- and long-term psychological problems owe more to the attitudes that patients form in the period immediately following their heart attack (Naismith et al 1979), and to their pre-existing psychological status (Cay et al 1972), than to the severity of their heart attack, medical complications or the presence of symptoms (Mayou, Foster and Williamson 1978a, Naismith et al 1979).

The applicability of all these findings to female heart attack victims is indicated by the results of several studies, most of which focused primarily on some other aspect of care, but all of which indicate that women may suffer higher levels of distress than men following heart attack. For example, an Indian study ($n = 80$) found that female heart attack victims expressed higher levels of death anxiety than did males, and higher levels than other patient groups (Kumar, Mohan and Nirmala 1987). An Australian study ($n = 120$: 93 men, 27 women) corroborated these findings by showing that female heart attack victims expressed more state anxiety than males on transfer from CCU (Byrne and Whyte, 1983). An Irish study ($n = 264$: 208 men, 56 women) confirmed women's greater psychological distress with anxiety, depression and low self-esteem four days after their heart attack (Guiry et al 1987).

Another large-scale study ($n = 338$: 254 men, 84 women) demonstrated significantly higher anxiety levels in women than among men admitted to a British CCU, and linked these high anxiety levels with fatal cardiac arrests in both men and women in the period prior to their discharge from hospital (Vetter et al 1977).

Resumption of Work

Another measure of poor psycho-social adjustment is the unnecessary failure of heart attack victims to return to work, i.e. where failure to return cannot be justified medically. This has been variously estimated at 10–50 per cent but, even among those who do not return to work, there is evidence of reduced satisfaction and performance (Cay et al 1972). In either event, unfavourable psychological and socio-economic consequences are liable to occur in the long term (Wishnie, Hackett and Cassem 1971).

A classic, albeit dated, study by Wynn (1967) followed 400 men for two years after their heart attacks. There was a widespread belief among subjects that the stressful nature of their jobs, either physical or emotional, was the cause of their heart attack in the first place. This belief was usually false, but nevertheless resulted in unnecessarily prolonged unemployment and inactivity causing increased anxiety, decreased security and decreased self-esteem. A similar though smaller study (Wishnie et al 1971) showed that, of the total number of subjects who were advised to resume employment, 46 per cent had failed to do so at six months. Furthermore, even those who did return to work showed considerable reluctance and anxiety about doing so. A study by Mayou et al (1978a) showed a delayed return to work at six months in 60 per cent of those previously employed, though 92 per cent had resumed by one year ($n = 100$).

Thus, although the percentage of those eventually returning to work may be high, unnecessarily long delays accompanied by anxiety are to be considered harmful. All three of the above studies, along with numerous others, confirm that the predictive value of medical factors such as severity of the attack and the presence of symptoms are, at best, about equal to psycho-social factors in determining the likelihood of return to work. These psycho-social factors relate mainly to negative attitudes which are formed during the first hours and days following heart attack, and which are amenable to influence by professional staff and relatives. For example, a study by Naismith et al (1979) showed that counselling and health education applied to a sample of 143 men resulted in a significantly earlier return to work.

Data on women are particularly scarce in this area since they tend to develop heart disease about ten years later in life than men, with a sharp increase after the menopause (Wenger 1985). With retirement at 60 in women, therefore, only a minority are still working outside the home when they have their first heart attack. However, two studies which will be described later indicate that, where women did work outside the home prior to their heart attack, their delay in returning to work was longer than that of men.

Quality of Family Relationships

One area in which women have received abundant research attention is in their role as spouses of male heart attack victims. It appears that wives suffer as much emotional distress as their husbands, and that heart attack affects the functioning of the whole family.

Skelton and Dominian (1973) studies 65 wives and described their initial response as a grief reaction characterised by: numbness, panic, insomnia, anorexia, anxiety and depression. They suffered feelings of guilt, as though they were in some way to blame for the heart attack, and developed various psychosomatic symptoms. The findings of Mayou et al 1978b) were very similar, with 38 per cent of wives suffering moderate or severe distress while their husbands were in hospital ($n = 82$). Wives also find the period following their husband's discharge to be particularly stressful, and continue to experience distress for at least a year (Skelton and Dominion 1973, Mayou et al 1978b, Hentinen 1983).

Mayou et al (1978b) found that, following their heart attack, 67 per cent of husbands decreased their leisure activities and 65 per cent undertook fewer household chores such as gardening and decorating. This obviously had implications for wives, who tended to take over heavy chores around the house, and decrease both work and leisure activities outside the home. Both this study and the Skelton and Dominian study capture the interpersonal tension which so often occurs as husbands become increasingly dependent and irritable. They often feel resentful, frustrated and humiliated at their changed role within the family and at watching their wives do 'men's jobs', often not to their own standards. Meanwhile, wives become over-protective and fearful of upsetting their husbands. They try hard to suppress any feelings of grievance or hostility for fear of upsetting their husband and precipitating another attack, and this inevitably leads to resentment and tension.

Studies vary in the amount of marital disharmony reported. For example, Wishnie et al (1971) report that all 18 couples studied showed a steady and eroding conflict, largely stemming from confused and discrepant understandings of one another's roles in the rehabilitation process. However, Mayou et al (1978b) found that only 20 per cent of marital relationships worsened and 25 per cent of couples reported improved relationships due to a lasting re-evaluation, a cessation of taken-for-grantedness and a consequent increase in tolerance and consideration.

Most studies support the conclusion that the extra strain of the heart attack leads to deterioration in a large number of marriages, and that a smaller but none the less significant number of relationships are characterised by increased closeness and commitment. Studies also agree that the marital outlook is better if the wife maintains her outside work and leisure commitments.

Sexual Activity

Although notoriously difficult to measure for a variety of reasons, and although sometimes confounded by the effects of medication, ageing and penile atherosclerosis, the research evidence indicates very clearly that sexual activity frequently undergoes a decline following heart attack, and that this decline is usually unconnected with biomedical factors.

In the Mayou et al (1978b) study, for example, twelve months after heart attack 25 per cent of men reported reduced frequency of sexual intercourse, 20 per cent reported less satisfaction and around 50 per cent reported no change ($n = 82$). In the Skelton and Dominian (1973) study, of those who were sexually active prior to their heart attack ($n = 38$): 29 per cent reported reduced frequency; 8 per cent reported cessation; 50 per cent reported no change; and 8 per cent reported increased frequency attributed to the husband's increased libido. A comparative study by Hellerstein and Friedman (1970) confirms the above, with 58 per cent of subjects reporting a reduction in frequency or complete cessation of sexual activity six months after the attack ($n = 48$) and, as regards quality ($n = 44$), 52 per cent reporting no change, 25 per cent a deterioration and 23 per cent an improvement.

Although, as we have come to expect, most studies of post-coronary sexuality have been carried out on men (e.g. Jones Watts 1976, Cooper 1986), there are two notable exceptions to this, each of which approaches the issue from a different perspective.

The first of these (Papadopoulos et al 1980) was a study of 100 wives of heart attack patients, all of whom were sexually active prior to their heart attack. The study showed that, following discharge from hospital, all wives had concerns about the advisability of sexual activity. Seventy-six per cent of couples finally resumed sexual activity within three years: 49 per cent with reduced frequency; 46 per cent to pre-morbid levels; and 5 per cent with increased frequency due to emotionally closer relationships.

The second study (Papadopoulos et al 1983) focused upon 130 female patients following their heart attack. Of those who were sexually active prior to their heart attack, 30 per cent expressed sexual concerns in relation to safety, quality of sex, or whether they would still be attractive to their husbands. In the absence of adequate advice, which is a common feature of all research in this area, the women were uncertain how long they should wait before resuming sex. In the event, however, 73 per cent had resumed at eleven weeks, 23 per cent did not resume due to loss of libido, fear or their husband's fear and 44 per cent reported decreased frequency.

Two Previous Comparative Studies

Having presented an overview of the literature on men's psycho-social adjustment following heart attack, and included what piecemeal and fragmented evidence is available on women, two studies which set out specifically to compare men and women will now be discussed.

The first of these was conducted by Stern, Pascale and Ackerman (1977) who compared a group of 13 women and 55 men as they recovered from their heart attacks. Subjects were followed from their admission to CCU until one year after their heart attack, and a range of psychological constructs were measured using well-established instruments. Overall, the findings confirm previous studies in that females had a much more difficult rehabilitation than males. They suffered a relatively high incidence of death, medical complications and readmission to hospital as well as greater psycho-social morbidity. Unmarried women, i.e. widowed, single or divorced, suffered a particularly high mortality rate.

After one year 80 per cent of women suffered from anxiety and/or depression compared with only 18 per cent of men, and women suffered significantly more social and marital difficulty. On average, women took longer to return to work, longer to resume sexual activity, and were less likely to return to their former levels of activity in both of these areas. Married women complained that their husbands tended to be over-protective, thus reinforcing feelings of inadequacy.

Women had high Type A scores, were very much orientated toward work-related goals and tended to displace intrapersonal tensions into the work arena. This typical Type A coping strategy was disturbed when heart attack forced them to slow down and face their personal problems.

The second comparative study was conducted by Boogard in 1984 and made a useful contribution to the literature by virtue of its ideas, rather than its results. Boogard hypothesised that psycho-social recovery following heart attack would be related to the individual's sexual self-concept or sex role orientation, i.e. whether they viewed themselves as being masculine or feminine. In order to test this hypothesis Boogard interviewed her subjects 3–6 months following their heart attack. Although the sample was very small ($n = 20$: 10 men, 10 women), and the results were not subjected to statistical analysis, Boogard's findings do show male–female differences, many of them along the lines we have come to expect: females delayed the resumption of sexual activity and the return to work for longer than men; they were less likely to attend rehabilitation classes; and resumed household chores earlier than males, and earlier than was considered advisable.

Although the families of all patients did perceive them as ill, and did not expect an early resumption of normal roles, females seemed to view their illness differently. Unlike males, they resisted help around the house and felt guilty about being unable to perform fully all their usual household activities and having to rely on others for help. Women apparently felt compelled to resume their household tasks, perhaps not understanding the high energy requirements of housework or perhaps not even regarding it as work. As Pinneo (1984) points out, women cannot get away from their (house)work in the same way as men can.

Perhaps there are pressures immanent within the family structure which urge women to resume their household chores whatever the verbal rhetoric may be, or perhaps the difference in womens' perception of their illness is a reflection of the societal view of CHD as a man's disease. Boogard (1984) suggests that there is a link between this compulsion to resume work and sex role orientation, with traditionally feminine women feeling urged to resume their homemaker/wife/mother roles as soon as possible.

Boogard's results confirm that women have a more difficult psycho-social recovery than men, but go further by offering an explanation related to sex role orientation and family dynamics. However, it was a very small study and there was no attempt to objectively measure sex role orientation or demonstrate an association with psycho-social outcomes. Thus, although the Boogard (1984) and the Stern et al (1977) studies have produced findings which are broadly consistent, and which agree with the fragments of evidence gleaned from more general studies, it is clear that much more research is needed in order to illuminate the problem and offer nursing prescriptions. The following study was intended as a small contribution.

A Comparative Study into Psycho-social Adjustment Following Heart Attack in Men and Women

Research Design

The study was based upon two hypotheses:

1. Women will experience a different psycho-social recovery from heart attack than will men.
2. Unfavourable psycho-social adaptation will be positively related to strength of sex role orientation in both men and women.

The first hypothesis is justified by the previous research that exists. The second hypothesis is derived from Boogard's ideas about sex role orientation.

According to Rogers's Self Concept Theory, the most fundamental human drive is to maintain and enhance our self concept (Rogers 1951). If, therefore, a highly masculine man has come to view himself as tough, efficient, self-reliant and instrumental, but is temporarily unable to act in that manner due to a disabling heart attack, then it would seem logical that he might suffer excess psychological discomfort.

If that is the case, then it may also be logical to suppose that women are in some way protected from CHD by their femininity, or rather by their lack of masculinity. However, women have their own self concepts and, within this, their own sex role orientation. It may be that women who are high in femininity are at particularly high risk of psycho-social morbidity following heart attack, as is the case in women following hysterectomy (Webb 1982). Women with a traditionally feminine sex role orientation have a strong self-concept of being a homemaker, the centre of the family, the nurturer, and so on. They expect to look after the family and provide stability and security both through the physical tasks of homemaking and through the conduct of affective interpersonal relationships (DeGregorio and Carver 1980).

Thus, it was hypothesised that individuals who are highly masculine or highly feminine will suffer greater psycho-social morbidity.

A correlational design was used whereby relationships were explored between variables which were identified in the literature search as having potential relevance. The independent variables identified included: age; sex; trait anxiety; sex role orientation; and so on. The dependent variables were: mood state; resumption of work; marital quality; and the resumption of sexual activity. The purpose of the study was to explore the effects of the independent variables upon the dependent variables.

Research Methods

Subjects were randomly approached when they attended post-coronary rehabilitation classes at one of two centres. The only inclusion criterion was a medical diagnosis of heart attack, though one of the ethics committees concerned also insisted on a lower age limit of 18. A final sample of 40 subjects was acquired: 19 women and 21 men. They varied in age between 41 and 74 with a mean of 56. Subjects were assured of confidentiality and were offered the option of using a pseudonym.

A total of four data collection instruments were used. The first was a 'homemade' questionnaire, which was mainly for the collection of biographical information. The second questionnaire was the Beck Depression Inventory or BDI (Beck et al 1979) which has been used extensively over the years with a variety of client groups, including medical patients. The third questionnaire was the State Trait Anxiety Inventory or STAI (Spielberger et al 1980). This test has also been used extensively on normal, medical, surgical, psychosomatic and psychiatric patients. The fourth questionnaire was the Golombok–Rust Inventory of Marital State (GRIMS) which was recently developed in the UK in order to assess the general quality of the relationship between heterosexual couples who may be either married or living together. The authors state that the test is suitable for investigating the impact of psycho-social or medical factors on a relationship (Rust et al 1988).

The fifth and final questionnaire was the Bem Sex Role Inventory (BSRI) which was originally developed in 1974 but revised in 1981 (Bem 1981). The development of this test represents a fundamental reconceptualisation of sexuality, whereby psychological androgyny replaces the concept of masculinity and femininity existing at opposite ends of a single bipolar continuum. The concept of androgyny constitutes a rejection of the notion that masculinity and femininity are mutually exclusive, and replaces it with the possibility of individuals possessing both (or neither) masculine and feminine qualities simultaneously. It was used in this study in order to measure the extent to which subjects saw themselves as conforming to traditional sex roles, i.e. their sex role orientation.

Data were then organised, categorised and encoded before loading for computer analysis by the Statistical Package for Social Sciences (SPSS) program. This program described and tabulated the data, and performed basic descriptive statistics, including measures of dispersion, central tendency and frequency distributions. The package was then programmed to conduct Pearson's Product Moment Correlations in order to explore the presence and strength of associations between all the variables. Following this, multiple regression analysis was performed in order to estimate the extent to which individual independent variables contributed to each of the dependent variable measures.

Findings

Independent variables

The sample was fairly homogeneous. All subjects except one were married or cohabiting (one was widowed), and all except one were white Caucasians. The only independent variables which may have influenced the findings were length of stay in hospital, the time elapsed since discharge from hospital and sex role orientation.

As regards the first point, correlations showed that women were detained in hospital significantly longer than men. This would seem to indicate a slower physical recovery or the presence of medical complications. Indeed, we know from previous studies (such as Wenger 1985) that women tend to suffer greater mortality, greater morbidity, more complications and a poorer response to treatment during their time in hospital following heart attack, though the Stern et al (1977) study indicates that womens' medical conditions did not justify this conclusion.

Another possibility is that women stayed in hospital for longer for psychological reasons. It may be that women's heart attacks are simply perceived as being more serious, i.e. by the patients themselves and/or by the medical staff, and more caution exercised in rehabilitation. If such an over-cautious approach were to exist, then this could reinforce negative feelings, thoughts and expectations in the patient and have a deleterious effect upon psycho-social recovery.

As regards the time elapsed since discharge, there was considerable variation in this, mainly because of a few extreme results, and the median and mode, both 13 weeks, are the most representative measures.

Masculinity was widely distributed between the sexes, perhaps indicating a high level of Type A characteristics among these female heart attack victims, but there was a positive correlation between femininity and female sex and a negative correlation of the same magnitude with male sex. The extent to which this may reflect a social desirability effect among men who did not view themselves as having feminine traits, or who would not admit to them, remains unknown. If such inhibitions do exist, however, they appear to be restricted to male subjects.

Mood state

BDI results show that 27 per cent of the sample were suffering from mild to severe depression. This correlated strongly with both state and trait anxiety. State anxiety scores were higher among younger subjects, something which previous studies have found (Rosen and Bibring 1966), and they were higher in women than men. Once again, this may indicate that the men experienced lower levels of subjective anxiety, or that they were reluctant to admit the full extent of their anxiety.

State and trait anxiety scores were strongly correlated, and multiple regression analysis indicated that they each made the major contribution in variations in the other. Surprisingly, however, trait scores were higher than state, meaning that patients were less anxious following their heart attack than they were formerly. If this finding is valid, then it may be due to the fact that both rehabilitation schemes relied heavily on anxiety reduction techniques including counselling, relaxation techniques and exercise.

Resumption of work

Of those subjects who worked outside the home prior to their heart attack (n = 26), two subjects returned to work only after an excessive delay and a further five subjects did not return at all, thus giving a total of seven (37 per cent) late or non-returners.

If any of the subjects were unable to return to work for medical reasons, it seems unlikely that their GP would have deemed them fit to participate in an exercise-based rehabilitation programme; it is reasonable, therefore, to assume that almost all the remaining non- and late returners were incapacitated primarily by psycho-social factors.

Interestingly, females were more likely to receive help from their partner than were males. This conflicts with Boogard's findings, but may still be consistent with her sex role orientation theory. It may be that men saw themselves as being tough, autonomous and independent, thus making it difficult for them to accept help with traditionally masculine chores around the house. Conversely, women may be seen as dependent, in need of protection and looking after.

Previous research indicates that having an over-protective partner is unhelpful in this situation, and the results of this study showed that 15 subjects (38 per cent) regarded their partner as being over-protective ($n = 40$). There were no sex differences.

Marital quality

Ten subjects (26 per cent) had severe or very severe marital problems. There was a positive correlation between those subjects who scored high on the GRIMS questionnaire and those who reported a deterioration in their relationship in the homemade questionnaire.

Contrary to the findings of most previous studies, more subjects reported that their marriage had improved following their heart attack compared with the number reporting a worsening, 17 subjects (44 per cent) compared with eight (21 per cent) ($n = 39$). Although previous studies have reported mixed results, on the whole, they have shown that more couples suffer a decline than enjoy an improvement in their general relationship.

Further, high GRIMS scores were positively correlated with the length of delay in resuming sexual intercourse. It may be that the marital relationship deteriorated following heart attack and, as part of this, the sexual aspect of the relationship also deteriorated. This is supported by the results of the homemade questionnaire.

Resumption of sexual activity

Several items in the homemade questionnaire addressed the issue of resuming sexual activity. Of the total sample, 35 subjects were sexually active prior to their heart attack and 29 of them reported that they had resumed sexual activities, though the time elapsing before this resumption varied considerably. Six subjects (17 per cent) reported that they had not yet resumed sex and, importantly, five of them were women. Furthermore, all six had been discharged from hospital for at least eight weeks and were, therefore, well past the point at which professional staff recommend a resumption. If those subjects who failed to resume sex are added to those who suffered excessive delay, then we have a total of 20 subjects, i.e. 57 per cent, who underwent unnecessary and potentially harmful delay in resuming their sex life, or who ceased altogether. Other subjects reported a reduction in frequency and occasionally in enjoyment.

Delayed resumption of sex also correlated with female sex and with femininity. Femininity was the only independent variable which emerged from multiple regression analysis as being predictive of the resumption of sex. Furthermore, subjects with high femininity scores tended not to resume sex at all. The generally poor sexual outlook among women is consistent with previous studies, though no previous study has examined the effects of femininity.

General comments

I am confident that greater significance could have been achieved if data were collected from a larger sample within a set time range following heart attack. Another factor which probably reduced significant morbidity measures is that the sample was self-selected and was undergoing therapy, thus introducing a variety of motivational, behavioural and therapeutic variables which may not otherwise exist. Another methodological deficiency lies in the limitations inherent in any correlational design whereby statistical techniques are used to show the presence and strength of relationships between variables, but do not establish the direction of these relationships. However, the study did enjoy considerable internal and external consistency.

Nursing Implications

We can conclude that there probably are significant sex differences in the psychological impact of heart attack, especially in older and single women, though the current state of knowledge does not offer nurses much guidance. It would be a mistake to assume that women's needs and problems are simply the same as men's, so until we know more we must approach each patient individually, bearing in mind the fragments of information and the ideas which are set out above. The following section will set out a few pointers which stem from the literature, and will locate them within the framework of the nursing process.

Assessment

It is reasonable to expect higher anxiety levels among female patients, though we have no grounds to anticipate the source or nature of that anxiety. Nurses therefore need to assess women's anxiety carefully by observing their behaviour, interpreting their vital signs and by asking them about their concerns. It may be that women will be more open about their fears than men.

We do not know what coping strategies women might use to deal with the stress of heart attack, but we know from the research on men and on women with other health problems that denial is an effective strategy in the early stages, provided that it does not interfere with medical treatment. We should therefore assess the extent to which women have accepted the reality of their situation. Denial is frequently evident only at a very subtle level, and nurses will need to question and listen carefully in order to detect it. Other coping strategies include information-seeking, and nurses need to be aware of important individual differences in the amount of information patients want. Social support is widely reported as having health benefits (e.g. House 1981) but female heart attack victims may no longer have a partner due to their greater longevity.

The literature on men is very clear that patients' early attitudes to heart attack are critical in influencing future psycho-social health. These attitudes are highly susceptible to influence by health care workers, and careless comments about, for example, heart failure can result in undue pessimism. Spouses are also very important in shaping attitudes, so nurses need to ensure that they understand the importance of an optimistic approach which assumes the patient will return to a full and normal life. The reaction of spouses should also be assessed since they themselves may suffer considerable distress and need support.

Nurses should also try to assess the extent to which self-concept has been damaged by the heart attack. This may be demonstrated in patients' verbal behaviour or may need to be elicited by careful questioning. For example, male patients frequently give cues about their threatened sexuality, and these can be followed up by incorporation into their care plan.

Planning

We know from research that post-coronary patient teaching which is planned is more likely to be effective than purely opportunistic teaching (e.g. Milazzo 1980), so all teaching and counselling should be written into the care plan.

During the first 24 hours or so, this should be directed mainly at anxiety reduction, but subsequently will involve information about risk factor modification and discussions about coming to terms with what has happened. It is clear from the plethora of research in other fields that such teaching and counselling should be planned to involve the patient's partner.

If the patient is in outside employment, the welfare officer or occupational health nurse should be notified, and encouraged to visit the patient at the earliest opportunity. This will help to foster positive attitudes and expectations about the future.

Care planning should include community follow-up, and where there is no cardiac rehabilitation scheme, nurses should consider initiating such a scheme.

It may well be that NHS Trusts will see this as a quality issue and support the scheme, though funds are also available from charitable organisations and from industry.

Naturally, the patient herself should be involved in care planning, and planning for the future can be very effective in avoiding pessimism and excess caution.

Implementation

Counselling should begin as soon as the newly admitted patient has stabilised in order to encourage an optimistic and positive attitude during the crucial first hours and days following admission, thus helping to avoid unnecessary invalidity. It should include explicit guidance on the resumption of physical activity, including sex, in order that couples should be quite clear about when it is safe, and indeed advisable, to resume. Euphemisms and vagaries need to be replaced by facts and applied examples, such as the energy expenditure involved in specific household tasks. This should be individualised by reference to the woman's particular life-style and interests, etc.

Nurses need to understand that some women will have traditionally feminine sex role orientations, and there may be pressures on them to quickly fall back into their role as homemaker and nurturer, etc. Other women, perhaps the 'new women' referred to earlier, may be pursuing a professional career, may have acquired Type A characteristics (traditionally associated with masculinity) and have different counselling needs. In both cases they may suffer excess distress.

Following discharge, nurses involved in rehabilitation schemes should be aware that women are poor attenders compared to men (e.g. Oldridge et al 1980, McGee and Horgan 1992), and there may be many reasons for this. One factor which I have observed is that exercise regimes are sometimes geared more to men than to women, with emphasis on weight training, power cycling, press-ups, etc., rather than (say) aerobic dance and movement to music. Research has demonstrated the importance of exercise for strengthening self concept, lifting depression and alleviating anxiety (e.g. Erdman and Duivenvoorden 1983, Taylor et al 1985).

Rehabilitation schemes should not be restricted to risk factor teaching and exercise, important as they are, but should include opportunities for patients and their partners to talk about mood changes, work, family relationships, and so on. Stress management techniques and relaxation training, including the modification of Type A behaviour, may result in a more favourable psycho-social and biomedical outlook (Friedman et al 1984). It is also important to facilitate mixing with other couples, from whom a good deal of support and reassurance can be obtained. There is now a growing body of literature to guide nurses working in this area (e.g. Thompson 1990, Bennett 1993), though most of it still focuses on male patients.

Conclusion

If nurses really are independent practitioners with a unique and holistic role, and not merely the technical agents of medical staff, then they should set about defining that role. They should lay claim to the territory described above and establish themselves as *the* primary agents of psycho-social care.

There is no better example of this than the field of cardiac nursing, whether in hospital or community settings, where there is considerable scope for nurses to use their psychological skills, and where there is a tremendous care gap to be filled. An important part of this care gap is sexuality, and nurses must grasp the nettle of their own discomfort in order to help heart attack patients to deal with their attitudinal and emotional needs, thus preventing much unnecessary psycho-social morbidity.

References

Bartley M, Farrant W and Russell J (1986) *Women's Health and Heart Disease*. London: Women's Health Information Centre, Broadsheet Number 15.

Baxter S (1975) Psychological problems of intensive care: 2. *Nursing Times*, 9 January, 63–65.

Beck A T, Rush A J, Shaw B F and Emery G (1979) *Cognitive Therapy of Depression*. New York: Guilford Press.

Bem S L (1981) *Bem Sex Role Inventory Professional Manual*. Palo Alto: Consulting Psychologists Press Inc.

Bennett P (1993) *Counselling for Heart Disease*. Leicester: British Psychological Society.

Boogard M (1984) Rehabilitation of the female patient after myocardial infarction. *Nursing Clinics of North America*, **19**, 3, 433–440.

Burke R J, Weir T and Duwors R E (1979) Type A behaviour of administrators and wives' reports of marital satisfaction and well being. *Journal of Applied Psychology*, **64**, 57–65.

Byrne D G and Whyte H M (1983) State and trait anxiety correlates of illness behaviour in survivors of myocardial infarction. *International Journal of Psychiatry in Medicine*, **13**, 1, 1–9.

Cay E L, Vetter N, Philip A E and Dugard P (1972) Psychological status during recovery from an acute heart attack. *Journal of Psychosomatic Research*, **16**, 425–435.

Chesney M A and Rosenman R H (1980) Type A behaviour in the work setting. In Cooper C L and Payne R (eds) *Current Concerns in Occupational Stress*. London: Wiley.

Cooper A J (1986) Sexual dysfunction following myocardial infarction in the male. *Stress Medicine*, **2**, 55–61.

Croog S H, Shapiro D S and Levine S (1971) Denial among male heart patients. *Psychosomatic Medicine*, **33**, 5, 385–397.

DeGregorio E and Carver C S (1980) Type A behaviour pattern, sex role orientation and psychological adjustment. *Journal of Personal and Social Psychology*, **39**, 2, 286–293.

Department of Health (1992) *The Health of the Nation – a Strategy for Health in England* (Cm 1986). London: HMSO.

Erdman R A M and Duivenvoorden H J (1983) Psychologic evaluation of a cardiac rehabilitation programme: a randomised clinical trial in patients with myocardial infarction. *Journal of Cardiac Rehabilitation*, **3**, 696–704.

Friedman M, Thoresen C E, Gill J J, Powell L H, Ulmer D, Thompson L et al (1984) Alterations of type A behavior and reduction in cardiac recurrences in postmyocardial infarction patients. *American Heart Journal*, **108**, 2, 237–248.

Gentry D, Foster S and Haney T (1972) Denial as a determinant of anxiety and perceived health status in the coronary care unit. *Psychosomatic Medicine*, **34**, 1, 39–44.

Greenglass E R (1982) *A World of Difference: Gender Roles in Perspective*. Toronto: Wiley.

Guiry E, Conroy R M, Hickey N and Mulcahy R (1987) Psychological response to an acute coronary event and its effects on subsequent rehabilitation and lifestyle change. *Clinical Cardiology*, **10**, 256–260.

Haynes S G and Feinleib M (1980) Women, work and coronary heart disease: prospective findings from the Framingham heart study. *American Journal of Public Health*, **70**, 2, 133–140.

Hellerstein H and Friedman E J (1970) Sexual activity and the post coronary patient. *Medical Aspects of Human Sexuality*, **70**, March, 987–999.

Hentinen M (1983) Need for instruction and support of the wives of patients with myocardial infarction. *Journal of Advanced Nursing*, **8**, 519–524.

House J S (1981) *Work Stress and Social Support*. Massachusetts: Addison-Wesley.

Jones Watts R (1976) Sexuality and the middle aged cardiac patient. *Nursing Clinics of North America*, **11**, 2, 349–359.

Khaw K T (1993) Where are the women in studies of coronary heart disease? *British Medical Journal*, **306**, 1145–1146.

Klein R F, Kliner V A, Zipes D P, Troyer W G and Wallace A G (1968) Transfer from a coronary care unit: some adverse responses. *Archives of Internal Medicine*, **122**, 104–108.

Kumar G, Mohan S and Nirmala S (1987) A study of death anxiety among heart attack patients. *Indian Psychological Review*, **32**, 1, 29–31.

Lloyd G G and Cawley R H (1978) Psychiatric morbidity in men one week after first acute myocardial infarction. *British Medical Journal*, 25 November, part 2, 1453–1454.

Lynch P and Oleman B J (1981) Mortality from coronary heart disease in the British army compared with the civilian population. *British Medical Journal*, **283**, 405–407.

Marmot M G and McDowell M E (1986) Mortality decline and widening social inequalities. *Lancet*, **ii**, 274–276.

Marmot M G, Rose G, Shipley M and Hammilton P J S (1978) Employment grade and coronary heart disease in British civil servants. *Journal of Epidemiology and Community Health*, **32**, 244–249.

Mayou R, Foster A and Williamson B (1978a) The psychological and social effects of myocardial infarction on wives. *British Medical Journal*, 18 March, part 1, 699–701.

Mayou R, Foster A and Williamson B (1978b) Psychological adjustment in patients one year after myocardial infarction. *Journal of Psychosomatic Research*, **22**, 447–453.

McGee H M and Horgan J H (1992) Cardiac rehabilitation programmes: are women less likely to attend? *British Medical Journal*, **305**, 283–284.

Milazzo V (1980) A study of the difference in health knowledge through formal and informal teaching. *Heart and Lung*, **9**, 6, 1079–1082.

Naismith L D, Robinson J F, Shaw G B and MacIntyre M M J (1979) Psychological rehabilitation after myocardial infarction. *British Medical Journal*, 17 February, 1, 439–442.

Oldridge M B, Lasalle D and Jones N L (1980) Exercise rehabilitation of female patients with coronary heart disease. *American Heart Journal*, **338**, 1366–1367.

Office of Population, Census and Surveys (1993) *General Mortality Statistics Series 1992*. London: OPCS.

Papadopoulos C, Larrimore P, Cardin S and Shelley S (1980) Sexual concerns and needs of the post-coronary patient's wife. *Archives of Internal Medicine*, **140**, 38–41.

Papadopoulos C, Beautmont C, Shelley S and Larrimore P (1983) Myocardial infarction and sexual activity in the female patient. *Archives of Internal Medicine*, **143**, 1528–1530.

Parsons T (1951) *The Social System*. New York: Free Press.

Petticrew M, McKee, M and Jones J (1993) Coronary artery surgery: are women discriminated against? *British Medical Journal*, **306**, 1164–1166.

Pinneo R (1984) Living with coronary artery disease. *Nursing Clinics of North America*, **19**, 3, 459–467.

Price L (1983) Epidemiology, medical sociology and coronary heart disease. *Radical Community Medicine*, **15**, 10–15.

Rogers C (1951) *Client Centred Therapy*. Boston: Houghton Mifflin.

Rosen I and Bibring G L (1966) Psychological reactions of hospitalised male patients to a heart attack. *Psychosomatic Medicine*, **28**, 808.

Rust J, Bennum I, Crowe M and Golombok S (1988) *The Golombok-Rust Inventory of Marital State Manual*. Nelson, Windsor: National Foundation for Educational Research.

Skelton M and Dominian J (1973) Psychological stress in wives of patients with myocardial infarction. *British Medical Journal*, 14 April, 2, 101–103.

Spielberger C D, Vagg P R, Barker L R, Donham G W and Westberry L G (1980) The factor structure of the state trait anxiety inventory. In Sarason I G and Spielberger C D (eds) *Stress and Anxiety*, 7. New York: Hemisphere/Wiley.

Steingart R, Packer M, Hamm P, Cogliangse M E, Gersh B, Geltman E H et al (1991) Sex differences in the management of coronary artery disease. *New England Journal of Medicine*, **325**, 4, 226–230.

Stern M J, Pascale L and Ackerman A (1977) Life adjustment post myocardial infarction. *Archives of Internal Medicine*, **137**, 1680–1685.

Taylor C B, Sallis J P and Needle R (1985) The relation of physical activity and exercise to mental health. *Public Health Reports*, **100**, 2, 195–202.

Thompson D R (1990) *Counselling the Coronary Patient and Partner*. London: Scutari Press.

Thompson D R, Webster R A, Cordle C J and Sutton T W (1987) Specific sources and patterns of anxiety in male patients with first myocardial infarction. *British Journal of Medical Psychology*, **60**, 343–348.

Toth J C (1980) Effect of structured preparation for transfer on patient anxiety on leaving the coronary care unit. *Nursing Research*, **29**, 1, 28–34.

Vetter N J, Cay E L, Philip A E and Stranger R E (1977) Anxiety on admission to the coronary care unit. *Journal of Psychosomatic Research*, **21**, 73–78.

Waldron I (1978a) Type A behaviour pattern and coronary heart disease in men and women. *Social Science and Medicine*, **12B**, 167–170.

Waldron I (1978b) Sex differences in longevity. *Proceedings from the Second Epidemiology of Ageing Conference*. Washington DC: Department HEW, NIH, NIA.

Webb C (1982) Body image and recovery from hysterectomy. In Wilson-Barnett J (ed.) *Recovery from Illness*, Chichester: Wiley.

Webb C (1985) *Sexuality, Nursing and Health*. Chichester: Wiley.

Wenger N K (1985) Coronary disease in women. *Annual Review of Medicine*, **36**, 285–294.

White J (1985) Coronary heart disease in women. *Precis Number 9, Winter 1985–6*. London: Education In Practice, Medical Tribune Group.

Wishnie H A, Hackett T P and Cassem N H (1971) Psychological hazards of convalescence following myocardial infarction. *Journal of the American Medical Association*, **215**, 8, 1292–1296.

Wynn A (1967) Unwarranted emotional distress in men with ischaemic heart disease. *The Medical Journal of Australia*, 4 November, 54, 847–851.

Chapter 10
Never-married Women's Health in Old Age
Christine Webb

Introduction

Women who have never married have formed an increasing proportion of the population of the UK since 1971, and this is a reversal of the trend between 1901 and 1971 (OPCS 1989). However, studies of women's health focus predominantly on its relationship to family and work roles in married women, and on comparisons of health and well-being in married women and men. When 'single' women are discussed writers often make no distinction between the never-married and the separated, divorced and widowed (see, for example, Verbrugge 1978, Rossi 1980, Briscoe 1982, O'Rand and Henretta 1983, Black and Hill 1984, Cooke 1985, Carp and Christensen 1986).

As a result, little is known about the health of never-married, nulliparous women. This may be because singlehood is a 'residual' or 'deviant' status in our society, with marriage being the statistical and culturally prescribed norm (Stein 1978).

Health

In relation to health, Verbrugge (1978) reports that in the USA unmarried women (widowed and never-married) have better health than the divorced and separated, and psychological well-being follows the same pattern. The major causes of morbidity in old age are painful musculo-skeletal problems, circulatory diseases and hearing impairments. Women have more genito-urinary problems, while emphysema is a greater cause of male morbidity. Work and leisure activities are limited mainly by arthritis, heart conditions and hypertensive disease, with visual and hearing problems also contributing. Hospital stays are related to malignant neoplasms, cerebrovascular disease and cardiovascular disease, in that order of frequency. Prostate problems occur for men and fractures for women. Heart disease is the principal cause of death for both sexes, with cancer and stroke in second and third place (Verbrugge 1986).

In the UK, health statistics are not given by marital status, but they do show that women over 65 report more long-standing illness and restricted activity, and have more general practitioner consultations and more out-patient hospital visits than men (OPCS 1987). This may be related to higher incidences of morbidity or to a greater willingness by women than men to report illness (Nathanson 1975). Patterns of illness in old age follow the social class inequalities found in early life, with morbidity being inversely related to social class.

Old age, therefore, will be a time of chronic physical ill health and disability for a significant proportion of women, with those aged over 75 years suffering the greatest impairment.

The prevalence of degenerative brain diseases such as Alzheimer's also increases with age, with 14 per cent of those over 65 years and 20 per cent of those over 85 years affected (Liptzin 1987). As women form the majority of this older age group, it is again mainly women who will suffer.

If organic brain disorders are excluded, then depression is identified as the most prevalent mental health problem of old age. However, the prevalence of all mental illnesses, including depression, is reported to decrease for those over 65 years (Gatz, Pearson and Fuentes 1983). The patterns of earlier life continue, with relatively more women than men diagnosed as depressed: Danello (1987) identifies depression as a disorder with special implications for older women.

The inter-relationship between physical and mental health is particularly pronounced in older age groups. There is greater somatisation of symptoms in depression, which frequently presents with physical problems such as insomnia, anorexia and fatigue, rather than with reports of mood change (Gatz et al 1983). Conversely, poor physical health may precipitate depression (Grau 1989). Indeed Sinnott (1985) reports that mental health symptoms in a sample of older people were related to health rather than to age *per se*, or to life stresses and conflicts, such as bereavement.

Marital Status and Health

A number of US studies have examined the relationship between marital status and health. Anson (1989) reports that marriage has consistently been found to be positively related to physical and psychological well-being, with married persons having lower mortality and lower morbidity rates than non-married persons. Within the non-married group it is the never-married women who appear to be healthiest, followed by the widowed. The divorced and separated have the highest acute and chronic morbidity rates, the most annual visits to a physician, and the highest hospitalisation rates (Verbrugge 1978, Anson 1989). Loss of a spouse, whether through death, divorce or separation appears to be associated with poorer health over time (Fenwick and Barresi 1981).

The limited data which relate to marital status and psychological well-being in women tend to reflect patterns of physical morbidity. In a US study of older women Hughes and Gove (1981) found that those who are married demonstrate better mental health than the unmarried. Among the unmarried, the never-married have the lowest prevalence of depression and the divorced and separated the highest (Keith 1987). There is some evidence, therefore, that marital status differentially affects the physical and mental health of older women.

Life Satisfaction

Most studies suggest that physical health is the most important correlate of life satisfaction in old age (Grau 1989). Verbrugge (1986) states that the quality of people's lives

> . . . depends greatly on the physical symptoms felt in daily life and the strategies individuals devise to care for them.

Carp and Christensen (1986) report that in older unmarried women, 'contentment' is associated not only with good health, but also with living in a safe, 'non-noxious' environment and having sufficient resources to entertain others.

Braito and Anderson (1983) discuss the conflicting evidence regarding marital status and reported happiness. Whereas some studies indicate that the never-married are less happy than the married and only slightly happier than the divorced and widowed, others, for example the early London study by Wilmott and Young (1960), report that never-married older people are happier than those who were married.

In general, older women identify the advantages of the single state as including the freedom to run their own lives and to do as they choose. These are balanced against the disadvantages of a lack of companionship and children, and general loneliness (Braito and Anderson 1983).

Seeking Health Care

The majority of studies depend on the self-reporting of symptoms and disability to determine prevalence. Indeed, as Wingard (1987) observes, sex differences in morbidity may reflect, at least in part, a greater willingness by women to report illness and disability. The subjective perception of health status is important as it not only influences psychological well-being and life satisfaction, but also shapes health behaviour.

Coulton and Frost (1982) suggest that it is older women's self-perception of their symptoms and needs, rather than other enabling and predisposing factors, that is of prime importance in prompting them to seek medical services. Similarly Engle and Graney's study of women over 60 years of age identifies perceived health, rather than physician assessment, as a significant predictor of health-care utilisation. The women in this study appear to define health mainly in terms of their ability to perform their usual daily activities and the ability to remain independent (Engle and Graney 1985). It would appear that health becomes salient when symptoms start to interfere with normal activities.

It is suggested that older women hold a personal norm of well-being and functional capacity against which they compare their current state. This norm comprises expectations and perceptions of both their own and their peers' health and functioning (Engle and Graney 1985). Support for this view comes from Ferraro, who discusses the 'normalization' of disability in older women. That is, if no additional limitations in function have occurred, then women with chronic disability evaluate their health more positively than women who have objectively less disability, but who have experienced a more rapid decline in function. Thus, 'holding one's own' becomes the norm (Ferraro 1985).

This raises the possibility of a high threshold of symptom toleration before help is sought and Rakowski et al (1988) state that older women tend not to report symptoms, particularly short-term discomforts and 'nagging', low-grade chronic conditions.

However, older women do consult their GPs more frequently than do older men (OPCS 1987) and although this may be beneficial, it may also increase older women's risk of iatrogenic, in particular drug-induced, disorders (Wingard 1987).

Previous use of services has been shown to be an important determinant of health care utilisation. In a longitudinal study Eve (1988) reports that it is established patterns of service use, rather than variations in impairment or perceived need, that determine subsequent service utilisation. Therefore, an older woman is more likely to use the system if she is familiar with it and knows how to access and evaluate it.

The 1981 *General Household Survey* (OPCS 1983) reveals that it is only a small minority of old people who receive support from statutory domiciliary services. The Home Help service is the most frequently used. However, there is some evidence that it is those who do not use the services who are in greatest need (Peace 1986).

Older women are more likely to perceive the need for mental health and recreational services, rather than personal care services. The converse is true for men (Coulton and Frost 1982). It can be speculated that this may be, in part, a reflection of traditional gender roles. That is to say, older women may find it particularly difficult to relinquish control over activities that tradition-ally fall within their domain. Health workers may share these perceptions, as there is evidence that men are more likely to receive personal care and home help services than are women with equivalent levels of disability (Peace 1986).

It appears, therefore, that older women in general demonstrate a high tolerance of physical symptoms and disability, but under-use services. Data relating to the influence of marital status on this behaviour are ambiguous, but marriage possibly has an inhibitory effect on both reporting symptoms and service utilisation.

Social Support

Social support factors such as living arrangements, family and friendship networks, and financial resources may act as mediating variables between marital status and health.

As women age they are increasingly likely to lose spouse, kin and friends through death. The impact of women's higher life expectancy is greatest for women over 75 years, 64 per cent of whom are widows, and the vast majority of these will live alone (OPCS 1983). Indeed, more elderly women live alone than any other population sub-group, and the proportion is increasing (Gatz et al 1983). Nearly 50 per cent of women in their late 70s and early 80s live alone (Peace 1986).

There is conflicting evidence regarding the consequences of living alone for the health and life satisfaction of older women. In general, involvement in social relationships is believed to have a positive effect on both physical and mental well-being. Prospective studies show that individuals who lack social ties at the time of initial measurement are more likely to die during the follow-up period (Umberson 1987). Marital and family relationships may be particularly salient social ties, but it cannot be assumed that living alone or being unmarried necessarily results in fewer meaningful social relationships.

Evidence to support living arrangements as a salient factor to the well-being of older women comes from Hunter et al (1979), who report that in a sample of both black and white older women, those who live alone have higher levels of social dysfunction, less life satisfaction and lower self-esteem than those who live with others. Significantly, they found no essential differences with respect to whether the person was living with a spouse or one or more other people.

It may be, therefore, that at least part of married women's health advantage arises from the positive effects of the presence of another person, rather than the married state *per se*. In this instance the proximate other is considered to play an important role in acting as confidante, which in turn helps to minimise the detrimental effects of the loss of both friends and physical function.

A potential implication of living alone, particularly within the context of a limited support network, is that if health does deteriorate to the point of not coping, then admission to a nursing or residential home may be the only option. In 1981, 75 per cent of those in residential homes were women (OPCS 1983). Women who live alone and those who never married are over-represented in the nursing home population relative to the general population (Danello 1987). Elderly men more frequently have a living spouse to care for them (Verbrugge and Wingard 1987).

Limited attention has been paid to the qualitative nature of the relationship between unmarried older women and those with whom they live. While some relationships may be supportive and positively affect well-being, others may have particular pressures. Hughes and Gove (1981) suggest that as families are usually focused on parents and children, they are not likely to include other unmarried adults easily. Fear of dependency and role reversal may put extra strain on the relationship (Gatz et al 1983).

Older women may also be acting as carers to elderly siblings, friends or even parents. The physical and emotional strains of caring for a dependant may negatively affect the older woman's own health.

Children are potentially an important source of social support to their parents as they age (Wan 1982). Shanas (1979) reports that 91 per cent of parents aged 65 years and over receive some help from their children in the form of gifts, help during sickness, financial aid or general advice. The impact of childlessness may be greatest in old age, particularly for those whose health is impaired. Those who are childless are more likely to be living alone and be socially isolated, although they are more likely to have close relationships with their siblings (Braito and Anderson 1983).

It may be that those with fewer family ties, such as the never-married, have larger networks of friends to compensate (Rubinstein 1987). In general, women are more likely than men to replace lost friendships and have a confidant (Gatz et al 1983). Babchuk (1978) identifies the never-married as being represented among both the socially isolated, in that they have no confidantes, but also among the very sociable. In addition, widows who have not developed many friendships outside the marriage may be vulnerable to the effects of social isolation on the death of their spouse.

Women who have limited social interaction and who do not have a confidante are more often depressed than those with confidantes and a higher level of social interaction (Babchuk 1978).

Economic Factors

In the UK the largest single group of those dependent on state benefit is older people, in particular the very old, and women are in the majority within this group (Payne 1991). Gatz et al (1983) state that:

Poverty may be the single most salient factor in the lives of too many old women now.

The limited resources of many older women reflect their concentration in lower-paid occupations, together with a history of discontinuous employment due to caring responsibilities. Thus they may have had less access to occupational pension schemes and have accrued limited pension credits (Peace 1986). The effect of economic constraints is to reduce options of life-style, particularly in the face of disability, when to a degree independence can be 'bought' through the purchase of aids and services.

The links between poverty and health have been well documented (Payne

1991). More specifically, regardless of marital status, lower income leads to lower levels of happiness and life satisfaction and higher reports of loneliness and worry.

Individual older women's financial circumstances will vary considerably independently of marital status. Anson (1989) suggests that the poorer health status of widows reflects access to fewer resources. The difference between widows' and other older women's health status disappears if socio-economic status is controlled.

Old age for many women, particularly the very old, is characterised by disability, isolation and poverty. Conversely, others may enjoy the freedom associated with retirement and the release from family obligations.

Summary of the Literature

It is older women's subjective perception of their health that is most salient to their well-being, and it is the impact of limited functioning in their daily lives that is of most significance to them. There is, however, a tendency to tolerate symptoms and under-utilise services.

There is evidence that marital status differentially affects older women's health. Physical and mental health may in turn not only influence each other, but also determine life satisfaction. It is married women who appear to experience better health than their unmarried peers, with the divorced and separated often faring worse than the widowed on measures of health status.

Social support resources may exert a potentially powerful mediating effect between marital status and health outcomes. Living arrangements are suggested to be of particular importance. Those who live alone and have few friends are particularly vulnerable. On the other hand, living with another person may be a source of strain or of support.

However, the evidence relating to the inter-relationship between marital status, social support resources, health and life satisfaction is often conflicting. This reflects, in part, the tendency for studies not always to discriminate between non-married states. Thus 'single' may include any combination of never-married, widowed, divorced and separated. In addition, a variety of scales have been used to measure health status and behaviour. Any meaningful comparison, therefore, between or generalisation from these studies is inevitably limited. Similarly, there has been little systematic measurement of life satisfaction in older women of different marital status.

Most of the research in this review emanates from the US and the population samples usually comprise white, urban, mainly middle-class women. The different health and social security systems in the US limit the relevance of these findings to UK populations. The effects of the interaction between marital status, ethnicity and rural or urban residence on older women's health have received little attention.

In conclusion, there has been little systematic investigation of the inter-relationship between parameters of health, life satisfaction, social support resources and marital status in older women. The mechanisms through which these variables impact on each other is not clear. There is the suggestion that some sub-groups, for example the never-married who live alone, may have unreported and undetected health problems which undermine the quality of their lives. If such 'at risk' groups can be identified, then screening procedures could be targeted more effectively and earlier intervention may not only limit current problems, but prevent further deterioration.

In view of the limited research on never-married women, I decided to conduct a small exploratory study to investigate health and coping in a sample of elderly spinsters.

Aims

The aims of the study were to investigate:

- perceptions of health and health care services;
- health care needs and service use;
- social support and its relationship to these factors

in single women over the age of 65 who had never been married and had had no children.

Methodological Considerations

The methodological approach of the study was that of reflexive ethnography (Hammersley and Atkinson 1983), and the method used was ethnographic interviewing. Reflexive ethnography is an approach developed from that used by anthropologists who have lived with and studied in depth the lives of groups of people, whether in their own or another culture. The reflexive aspect emphasises the importance of considering how the researcher affects and in turn is affected by the research experiences. The presence and actions of a researcher within a social group will clearly alter social processes and it is essential that readers are aware of this influence so that they are able to judge the validity of the research report. Reflexive ethnography is appropriate when studying a previously under-researched area where theory-testing is not possible and, in keeping with the tenets of the approach, the empirical aspects of the study will be reported using the first person (Webb 1992).

I hoped that the study would generate rich data, expressed and understood from the interviewees' perspectives, and that it would identify commonalities in the life histories and experiences of the women interviewed. My interview agenda was of necessity open-ended and, by focusing on a health history, I hoped that the women would identify for me what was important in their lives and health rather than my imposing preconceived ideas on them. I therefore saw them as participants and not as subjects of the research.

I planned to explain to participants that I was an experienced nurse with a particular interest in women's health, that the health of single women was an interesting but relatively unexplored topic, and that as a single woman approaching middle age myself I was particularly interested in learning from their experiences what I might expect for myself in the future.

Access to the sample was gained via two general practices, after obtaining the necessary ethics committee approval. I then wrote to each woman in advance explaining the study, and that her general practitioner (GP) had given her permission to approach her. At the bottom of the letter was a tear-off slip to be signed and returned in a stamped addressed envelope if she was prepared to be interviewed. On receipt of the replies I contacted women by telephone or by calling at the home to make an appointment. On arrival I handed each woman a 'visiting card' with the same design as the letterhead on which I had previously written to her.

Fifteen women were interviewed over a period of six months, with those from a housing estate being seen before those from a suburban area. Twenty-one women were approached, but two were married and had been mis-classified on the GP's register, one had died, and three did not reply to the letter. Interviews lasted between 45 minutes and two hours, were tape-recorded, and centred on the woman's health history and how she had coped with various health-related experiences. The latter were interpreted broadly to include family life, work and leisure, in so far as they related to health and social support. No further interviews were conducted when new data ceased to emerge, but the supply of interviewees from the two general practices was also close to exhaustion.

Data were analysed by playing the tape-recordings repeatedly and making verbatim notes of critical sections. As an experienced researcher I did not feel it necessary to transcribe all tapes. This is time-consuming and therefore costly, and I had not been successful in raising funds to support the study. It is difficult to obtain funding for qualitative research, and funders often expect small-scale exploratory work such as this to be carried out to test the feasibility of a larger study that may attract funding.

I listened to and made notes on the tapes concurrently with data collection so that I was able to identify emerging themes and use these in subsequent interviews to check their validity, while still pursuing the original scheme of using a health history to elicit information. As a result similar data were obtained from all women but also salient themes were explored and validated.

Women's Biographical Information

Ages ranged from 66 to 89, with a mean and median of 77. Three 'young elderly' were in their 60s and six participants were over 80 years of age. Six women living on the housing estate were interviewed, all of whom could be categorised as working-class because they had done manual work in factories. Of the nine women interviewed from the suburban area, one had previously done skilled manual work, three had been nurses of various types, two had done office work, and three had been employed in family shops and had taken these over when their fathers had retired. Of the last three, one had done book-keeping but the other two had done manual work, as a florist and a cycle repairer. In terms of occupational background, then, suburban interviewees were quite mixed in their background and economically their lives were very different, one typist living in rather straightened circumstances while the former family book-keeper and florist were 'comfortably off'.

In other ways the sample was surprisingly homogeneous, despite differing financial resources. All but three had lived with their parents in the parental home all their lives until the last parent died. Only the three 'nurses' (one nurse, one midwife, and one residential child care nursery nurse) had lived away because of their work and had never returned to live in the parental home. All 15 women were living alone and had been doing so for many years.

Contrary to expectations, none of the women had been involved in caring for aged parents except for a relatively short period. All those who had lived with their parents had moved to smaller accommodation after the parents' death.

Health

The kinds of conditions women reported were those to be expected in people of this age (Verbrugge 1986). Six women had arthritis, mainly affecting the knees, hips and feet. One was awaiting admission to hospital for hip replacement, and another was severely limited by an arthritic knee, which she had been told could not be treated by replacement surgery. She was reluctant to take medication for her pain because her mother had had a perforated gastric ulcer due to taking drugs for her arthritic hip. As with several women, her feet caused her the greatest trouble.

> The worst thing is my feet, I've got no flesh under the balls of my feet. I walk on the bones. I see old ladies with sticks and I see their faces and I think it must be their feet. I suppose I've worn them out.

In addition to five who were taking medication for heart conditions, current health problems included shingles, cataract (three women), Menière's disease, oesophagitis and hearing loss. All women could name at least two current health problems that were being treated or needed treatment. They were taking a variety of medications, and one was taking ten different substances. Only one had had a 'screening' visit from a practice nurse, and all others obtained repeat prescriptions by phoning or calling at the GP's surgery.

A striking feature of their past medical histories was that four of the 15 women had had 'nervous breakdowns' and had been treated with electro-convulsive therapy. One woman said:

I took an overdose in 1988 when I lost my mother. I didn't expect to wake up. I wouldn't do it again because I'd have to go to X hospital again – it's the worst hospital you can go in. It's a very bad experience. The hospital is very unkempt due to lack of funds . . . You see others who won't get better.

The hospital mentioned is a former workhouse which regularly features in local newspaper reports as suffering from under-resourcing, and discussions are in progress about its demolition and rebuilding on another site.

From one of the quotations already given it is clear that several women had idiosyncratic explanations for their illnesses. Many were taking multiple medications and had little or no idea what these were for: several asked me for explanations about their tablets. The one woman who had had a screening visit from a practice nurse asked me for advice about managing her incontinence. Not wanting to interfere with what might already have been suggested, I enquired what the practice nurse had said about this. However, the woman had not discussed the problems with the practice nurse, despite the fact that she felt that this was her principal health concern.

Support resources

When asked how they would manage if they were ill, women's replies revealed that their support resources were extremely limited and precarious. Most did not have any surviving relatives, and those with relatives lived too far away to seek help from them.

One woman who had had a stroke and suffered from arthritis had difficulty in getting out of her flat. She depended on her 80-year-old brother-in-law, who lived upstairs in the same block, to help her. He brought her lunch daily from a nearby community centre. She had no telephone. She had fallen in the flat some months earlier and broken her collar bone, but was unable to get any help until the following day when her brother-in-law called in.

Another who was housebound with severe arthritis had had a cholecystectomy when she was aged 70, a mastectomy at 82 and a lymph gland removed the following year. Following these operations, as well as her recent knee replacement, she had come home to her flat and been completely alone but for a neighbour who called in and did her shopping. She had a weekly home help. Three times in the past two years, youths had broken into her first floor flat while she was there. On the last occasion they had stayed for a long time, eating food from her kitchen and generally making a mess in the flat. She could do nothing but simply sit there and wait for them to go away. During the interview she asked me if I could try to do something about her curtains, which would not close properly, because she was afraid that people could see into the flat at night.

One participant said that if she was ill she would

just have to manage. I have to look after myself. I'd have to come down and let the dog out. A neighbour would do the shopping.

However, another, whose family had had a wholesale grocery business and who seemed financially secure, said that if necessary she 'would get a nurse in like we did for mother, I suppose'.

More typical was the reply that:

If I got ill – I don't know how I'd manage. I'd have to wait and see.

Maintaining Independence

Maintaining their independence was a major priority for all women, and they linked this with having been single and always managing their own lives. They expressed their feelings in different ways, some positively but others more negatively or resignedly:

I want to manage on my own without people looking after me . . . It's not what I've been used to . . . living close to people.

You've got to rely on yourself if you're going to get anywhere. If I'm going to stay out of a home I've got to rely on myself.

One woman, who had only a state pension and had been drawing on her savings for routine living expenses for several years, said:

You've got to keep going . . . I just scrape along.

Most participants were desperate not to have to 'go into a home'. A relatively well-off woman said:

I don't want to go into a home . . . I want to stay on my own as long as I can. I'd have to sell the house to pay to go into a home. I don't know if I'd get on with people.

Another, who visited such homes with a church group, based her views on knowledge of what she might expect:

I don't want to go . . . I'd have to be desperate. I think, oh my, I hope I never have to come. They all sit round looking at one another. The ones who are there all the time (in contrast to day patients) can't bring themselves to join in. When they get there, they lose all interest. They don't even want to get up because they've got no interests.

Only two viewed residential care as something that they might be able to accept, one putting it this way:

I accept that I'll have to go into a home. Some of the places are quite nice – others not. A friend who's 80 is in one and is very happy. I'm going there today for her 80th birthday. I've also been to Y home . . . I've accepted that that's what would happen . . . I'd have to go in somewhere.

As far as pastimes were concerned all women had now given up their past hobbies because of declining mobility and stamina. Three had formerly played golf and one had gone dancing twice weekly. The golf players now played bridge with the same friends, but going to church was the main social activity for several women. Reading and watching television were the most common pastimes for those who were unable to get out. These are, of course, solitary pursuits, and this was a source of regret to some:

Looking back I've been very fortunate. I've lived a full life. Of course it's very different now. I don't see many people.

I've been very blessed. I've had a good life. I've worked hard . . . But if you keep occupied, keep going . . . I don't worry about dying . . . I just get up in the morning and carry on. TV is a big help – it's part of my life. I used to think that was silly but I don't now. I get interested in it.

There was also a recognition that being single brought some advantages in old age because:

It's easier. You are used to managing if you've had nobody close to you. Some widows have been so dependent on the husband. Another friend could not bring herself to live alone – she went and lived with another friend.

Another said:

I like to be alone, that's the beauty of it. I've always coped and therefore I need less help. In marriage you've got to be prepared to sacrifice yourself completely and I'm not prepared to . . . I'd rather have my dog!

Mother–daughter Relationships

An unanticipated theme to emerge from the interviews was the strength of these women's relationships with their mothers. Twelve of the 15 had lived with their mothers until the latter's death, and often this period of co-residence had lasted for more than 20 years since the father had died. Although the mothers' deaths had taken place over 15 years before the interviews, the women obviously still felt very emotional about their relationships with their mothers. Whether the relationship had been positive or negative, it had had a profound and lasting influence and several interviewees cried as they told me about it.

To illustrate these mother–daughter relationships, two case histories will be presented to illustrate both negative and positive relationships, and how influences from childhood can have a lasting and pervasive effect on thinking and on daily living.

Case History 1

Miss B was 84 and she had lived with her mother 'like two sisters' from 1939 to 1967 when her mother died. Her father had died when she was a child and she had gone to live with her grandparents. Her mother remarried but this second husband also died and Miss B had returned to live with her mother. Mrs B had had a hysterectomy and two years later, aged 29, Miss B had one also and so they were able to share this and so many other experiences.

Miss B described herself as the tenant of the accommodation she shared with her mother, but it had been her mother who had taken all the decisions. Miss B accepted this because they were so close. She described her mother as 'a strong spirit but not physically strong', due a 'damaged throat from sucking a doll painted with lead paint when she was a child'. Miss B had always done the housework but her mother had done the cooking. Of her mother's death she said:

> When she died the biggest difference was not having a cooked meal ready when I came in. I lacked confidence in cooking. I could cook but she always told me what do do . . . I missed her . . . I came in and thought, 'I must tell my mother that' – but she wasn't there.

She explained how she had really only learned to cook after her mother died, and that after a few weeks she had realised that the house was becoming very untidy because nobody was tidying up and putting things away as her mother had done. She had to learn these basic housekeeping skills, as well as planning and budgeting and seeing that the bills were paid. Of the financial side of things, she commented:

> That was a bit grim. I was in a bit of a pickle when it was just my wage. I just had to sweat it out – I just learned the hard way.

Case History 2

Miss C was 81 and seemed very frail. She said that she had been healthy up to the age of 60, although she had been 'delicate' as a child following rheumatic fever which had left her with mitral valve damage. She had had a mastectomy 10 years earlier, but her main problem now was severe arthritis which meant that she was virtually chairbound.

As a child she had lived with her grandparents until she was 12 years old because her mother had been 'in service'. At the age of 12 she had been sent to live in a convent school and on leaving there had been in lodgings for four years until going to live with her mother in rented rooms. She had then lived with her mother continuously until the latter's death in 1973 at the age of 89.

Miss B had cared for her mother as she became older, but had continued in paid employment. She washed and dressed her mother and sat her in a chair. Her mother had behaved selfishly during this period, insisting that the home help spend time with her rather than doing the housework, so that Miss C had to do this too. Her mother had been unable to walk, but Miss C was not sure why this had been and seemed to be suggesting that her mother could have been more independent if she had wanted to be.

When her mother had died Miss C had been

Very sad. She had always had a chip on her shoulder. My brother died when he was 6 and she turned round and said 'I wish it had been her' (Miss C). After she died I found I had been born out of wedlock. She should have told me. I found out through a birth certificate. Other people knew, but not me. I kept thinking about hints, etc., on my father's side. They more or less pushed me out. I'd have liked to know. I thought she could have trusted me better. She was a good mother, but most of it was just duty.

Miss C then, like Miss B, had had a very strong attachment to her mother, but the relationship had not been of the same positive quality. The long years of her mother's resentment against her because she had become pregnant with Miss C before getting married still weighed very heavily, and Miss C cried as she told me her story. She had worked for some years in a children's nursery and said of this:

Some of the children I've looked after never knew their fathers – it didn't make any difference.

In saying this she seemed to be expressing the fact that it should not have made any difference to the way her mother had treated her, and the fact that it had done so was still a source of great distress to her.

Discussion

The study focused on a small convenience sample of never-married women in old age, all of whom lived alone and the majority of whom had spent their whole lives in the parental home until their parents died. The results are clearly not generalisable, but do raise issues for nurses. With the rise of geographical mobility it is possible that the numbers of similar women in the future will be small. However, such mobility may mean that elderly single women are even more isolated from kin support and from friendships they had been involved in when younger.

The particular cohort studied may be among the last of what has been termed a distinct 'social type' (Rubinstein 1987). Family patterns and lower levels of geographical mobility than today meant that women who did not marry tended to remain in the parental home for most of their lives. The case histories show that mother–daughter relationships retained an intensity that might have been transferred to a husband, had the women married. It is therefore not surprising that mothers' deaths constituted a major life event for these elderly daughters, and this conclusion matches that of Rubinstein (1987), who writes:

> There exist for some (never-married people) deep feelings of loss and abandonment upon the death of parents (who) were co-residents into mid- or late-life. Theirs is not an unfelt, lossless old age, a conclusion that might be inferred from a focus on the lack of marital bereavement.

Women in the study gave an impression of strongly defended independence in the face of multiple pathology and extremely precarious social support resources, as Evers (1985) also reports of her study of older women. They gained self-esteem from the fact that they had always coped for themselves and they continued to expect that they would do so. They were also keenly aware that others also expected them to manage, and some compared their position to that of widows, whom they perceived as seeking and getting more attention.

On the whole they led simple but contented lives, not dominated by concerns for their health or other matters. Several were in precarious financial circumstances. However, they appeared to have resolved past conflicts and mental health difficulties, and to face life on a day to day basis calmly and happily.

The 1981 *General Household Survey* (OPCS 1983) showed that very few old people receive support from statutory domiciliary services. As in the present study, home helps were the most frequent service used. Only one woman had meals on wheels, and none went to a lunch club.

The women who participated in this study resemble Evers' 'active initiators' in that they have invested 'energy in activities over and above their involvement in traditional women's work . . . right across the lifespan' (Evers 1983). While Evers' subjects were not all never-married women, her conclusion seems relevant to my participants. She suggests that in terms of formal support a different approach may be needed for these women, and that what is appropriate can only be judged on the basis of women's self-perceptions of their situations. Their apparent ability to cope may mask very fragile health and caring arrangements and, having coped for themselves throughout their lives, they may be particularly reluctant to ask for help.

Implications for Nurses

It is clearly important for community health workers to be aware of these women's potential special needs. A district nurse or practice nurse may be involved with or know about the death of the mother, and should anticipate the enormity of the loss caused to a never-married daughter by her bereavement. Bereavement support and counselling may be even more necessary than for widows who have a family of marriage around them, and Community Psychiatric Nurses may also have a role to play. Referral to a social worker or health visitor may be appropriate to help the woman to manage her finances and any change in housing arrangements that m. y be necessary.

Because their social support resources are likely to be limited, never-married women may be in greater need than some others of district nursing, home help and meals on wheels when they are acutely ill, discharged from hospital, or disabled on a more long-term basis.

Coulton and Frost (1982) conclude that those who do not use social services are those in most need. Their lack of contacts and social isolation militate against service use, whereas more gregarious and sociable people use such services more. On the basis of my study, this would be an important consideration for practice and other community nurses in respect of never-married elderly women. The fact that their social support resources are so limited may mean that they need referral to district nurses more readily than other elderly people who can depend on kin support, and they may need home nursing for longer periods. Information about reduced costs for installing a telephone may assist in lowering the risk of needing but being unable to call for help.

As far as health education and teaching about illness and its prevention and treatment are concerned, the poor knowledge and misunderstandings revealed by these women may not differ from those of others of similar age. However, they have fewer people to consult about health and illness, and community nurses can help by being aware of and filling their knowledge gaps.

When elderly never-married women are admitted to hospital they are likely to be particularly anxious to return home to independence. Hospital nurses can help them to achieve their goals by ensuring that adequate support services are arranged for their discharge.

Nurses in residential care settings need to be sensitive to the acute sense of privacy that never-married elderly women may have because they have lived alone for many years and are unaccustomed to and uneasy with the social routines and trivia of everyday living with others.

Conclusion

In a review of the literature on ever-single elderly women, Braito and Anderson (1983) begin their article by noting that 'we have no knowledge of current ever-single elderly women', and they conclude in the same vein that 'problems associated with being an ever-single woman and elderly may be widespread or insignificant; we do not know'. I hope that this small, exploratory study has indentified some of the special experiences and needs of the present cohort of never-married elderly women and some of the ways in which nurses, by being aware of their situations, can help them to maintain the independence and dignity that they value so much.

References

Anson O (1989) Marital status and women's health revisited: the importance of a proximate adult. *Journal of Marriage and the Family*, **51**, 185–194.

Babchuk N (1978) Aging and primary relations. *International Journal of Aging and Human Development*, **9**, 137–151.

Black S M and Hill C E (1984) The psychological well-being of women in their middle years. *Psychology of Women Quarterly*, **8**, 3, 282–292.

Braito R and Anderson D (1983) The ever-single elderly woman. In Markson E W (ed.) *Older Women: Issues and Prospects*. Lexington: Heath.

Briscoe M (1982) Sex differences in psychological well-being. *Psychological Medicine. Monograph Supplement 1*. London: Cambridge University Press.

Carp F M and Christensen D L (1986) Older women living alone. *Research on Aging*, **8**, 3, 407–425.

Cooke D J (1985) Social support and stressful life events during midlife. *Maturitas*, 7, 303–313.

Coulton C and Frost A K (1982) Use of social and health services by the elderly. *Journal of Health and Social Behaviour*, **23**, 330–339.

Danello M A (1987) Health concerns of older women. *Public Health Reports* (Supplement), **102**, 14–16.

Engle V F and Graney M J (1985) Self-assessed and functional health of older women. *International Journal of Aging and Human Development*, **22**, 4, 301–313.

Eve S B (1988) A longitudinal study of use of health care services among older women. *Journal of Gerontology*, **43**, 2, M31–39.

Evers H (1983) Elderly women and disadvantage: perceptions of daily life and support relationships. In Jerrome D (ed.) *Aging in Modern Society. Contemporary Approaches*. London: Croom Helm.

Evers H (1985) Frail elderly women. In Lewin E and Olesen V. *Women, Health and Healing. Toward a New Perspective*. London: Tavistock.

Fenwick R and Barresi C M (1981) Health consequences of marital status change among the elderly: a comparison of cross-sectional and longitudinal analyses. *Journal of Health and Social Behavior*, **21**, 106–116.

Ferraro K F (1985) The effect of widowhood on the health status of older persons. *International Journal of Aging and Human Development*, **21**, 1, 9–25.

Gatz C, Pearson C and Fuentes M (1983) Older women and mental health. Setting the stage. *Issues in Mental Health Nursing*, **5**, 1, 273–299.

Grau L (1989) Mental health and older women. *Women in the Later Years*, **14**, 304, 75–91.

Hammersley M and Atkinson P (1983) *Ethnography: Principles in Practice*. London: Routledge.

Hughes M and Gove W R (1981) Living alone, social integration and mental health. *American Journal of Sociology*, **87**, 1, 48–75.

Hunter K, Linn M W, Harris R and Pratt T C (1979) Living arrangements and well being in elderly women. *Experimental Aging Research*, **5**, 6, 523–535.

Keith P M (1987) Postponement of health care by unmarried older women. *Women and Health*, **12**, 1, 47–60.

Liptzin B (1987) Mental health and older women. *Public Health Reports*, **102** (Supplement), 34–38.

Nathanson C (1975) Illness and the feminine role. *Social Science and Medicine*, **9**, 57–62.

Office of Population Censuses and Surveys (1983) *Census 1981*. London: HMSO.

Office of Population Censuses and Surveys (1987) *General Household Survey*. London: HMSO.

Office of Population Censuses and Surveys (1989) *Social Trends 19*. London: HMSO.

O'Rand A and Henretta J C (1983) Women in middle age: developmental transitions. *Annals of the American Academy of Political and Social Science*, **464**, 57–64.

Payne S (1991) *Women, Health and Poverty*. Hemel Hempstead: Harvester Wheatsheaf.

Peace S (1986) The forgotten female: social policy and older women. In Phillipson C and Walker A (eds) *Aging and Social Policy: a Critical Assessment*. Aldershot: Gower.

Rakowski W, Julius M, Hickeky T, Verbrugge L M and Halter J B (1988) Daily symptoms and behavioural responses. Results of a health diary with older adults. *Medical Care*, **26**, 3, 278–295.

Rossi A S (1980) Lifespan theories and women's lives. *Signs*, **6**, 1, 627–635.

Rubinstein R L (1987) Never married elderly as a social type: re-evaluating some images. *The Gerontologist*, **27**, 1, 108–113.

Shanas E (1979) Social myth as hypothesis: the case of the family relations of old people. *The Gerontologist*, **19**, 3–9.

Sinnott J D (1985) Stress, health and mental health symptoms of older women and men. *International Journal of Aging and Human Development*, **20**, 2, 123–132.

Stein P (1978) The lifestyles and life chances of the never-married. *Marriage and the Family Review*, **1**, 1, 3–11.

Umberson D (1987) Family status and health behaviours: social control as a dimension of social integration. *Journal of Health and Social Behaviour*, **28**, 306–319.

Verbrugge L M (1978) Sex and gender in health and medicine. *Social Science and Medicine*, **12** (5A), 239–333.

Verbrugge L M (1986) From sneezes to adieu: stages of health in American men and women. *Social Science and Medicine*, **2**, 11, 1195–1212.

Verbrugge L M and Wingard D L (1987) Sex differentials in health and mortality. *Women and Health*, **12**, 2, 103–145.

Wan T (1982) *Stressful Life Events, Social Support Networks and Gerontological Health*. Lexington, Massachusetts: Lexington Books.

Webb C (1992) The health of single never-married women in old age. *Journal of Advances in Health and Nursing Care*, **1**, 6, 3–29.

Wilmott P and Young M (1960) *Family and Class in a London Suburb*. London: Routledge and Kegan Paul.

Wingard D L (1987) Health among older women in the United States. *Public Health Reports* (Supplement), **102**, 62–67.

Chapter 11
I Feel That I'm a Carer Now: Nurses' Working Lives
Mary Black

Introduction

The process of change is not just a sequence. It is a process fuelled by a variety of interpretations, each of which provides the spur to action, creates the vision and sustains the energies of those participants caught up in the process of change.

(Wilson 1992, 83)

The 'view from below' as expressed by nurses working on a Nursing Development Unit to me as a 'stranger' or non-nurse researcher is the focus of this chapter. I carried out an ethnographic study so that the voices of the nurses themselves could be heard, as they told me about the changes that have taken place in their unit since the early 1980s and the changes in their own working lives.

Histories of nursing often feature 'change as primarily the outcome-oriented pursuit of great and charismatic individuals' (Wilson 1992, 122), in the style of Florence Nightingale. The role played by managers and educationalists in initiating and sustaining improvements in nursing care in the elderly unit that I studied is discussed elsewhere (Black 1993a). This chapter will focus on the experiences of a group of nursing staff, including nursing auxiliaries, working in the care of the elderly unit in a district general hospital – traditionally a low status area of nursing work.

Twenty nursing staff who had worked in the Unit since the mid-1980s or for longer were interviewed between May 1991 and January 1992. Nine were Registered General Nurses (RGNs), of whom seven were sisters. Five enrolled nurses also took part in interviews, and six nursing auxiliaries. Eight worked on night duty and 12 on day duty.

All but one of the nurses interviewed were women. Most of them combined paid employment with a major share of domestic and childcare work, and as Dex (1991) suggests, it is 'impossible to understand life without work experiences and vice versa'. Therefore, after setting the scene, the chapter explores the ways in which women came into nursing and the social networks that link their home and work histories as a prelude to their descriptions of patient care and the satisfaction that they derive from their work. The discussion is drawn together by drawing links between improving the status of women's work and their own levels of self-esteem and pride and satisfaction in their work.

Setting the Scene

Defining Nursing as Women's Work

Gender divisions provided a justification for inequality between nursing and medicine in the mid-nineteenth century. Gamarnikow (1978) suggests that Nightingale saw the relationships between doctor, nurse and patient as similar to the family structure, with the doctor as the father figure, the nurse as the mother and the patient as the child. Gamarnikow (1978, 111) claims that nursing reformers reinforced the idea of nursing as suitable work for women:

They were motivated by a desire to open up non-industrial occupations for women: at the time, teaching was the only 'respectable' job available to women of bourgeois and petit-bourgeois origins who were forced, by adverse circumstances such as the lack or death of a husband or the lack of any inheritance to earn their own living.

The working patterns of married women have changed in the twentieth century, so that most combine paid work with family and domestic responsibilities at home. Joshi (1985, 75) refers to the limited range of jobs that most women do:

Women's employment has always tended to be concentrated in relatively few occupations which on the whole are not performed by men. The sex segregation of employment has changed little over the long run. Even in the 1980s women are concentrated in the caring professions and in service occupations.

James (1989) uses the concept of 'emotional labour' developed by Hochschild (1983) in a study of flight attendants on a US airline and, referring to the skills associated with emotional labour, claims:

The circumstances under which they are employed in the public domain may not only leave them unrecognised, but may use their low status in the domestic domain to define the equivalent paid work in the public domain as unskilled and therefore low paid.

Salvage (1992, 10) echoes this view:

> It is impossible to understand nursing without acknowledging its position as a female occupation doing archetypal 'women's work'.

However, these insights are not commonly shared within the nursing world. The perceptions of women as employees in this study were similar to those found by Cockburn (1991, 169) in a study of equal opportunity initiatives in four organisations:

> I was told over and again in the course of this research that women's lower pay and lower status at work is no more than incidental to the economic class interests of employers and to the career chances of male employees, that on the contrary it springs solely from the 'supply side' factor: women's inevitably domestic persona. These ideas are hegemonic in the sense that they appear as common sense truth to most men, and more significantly, to most women.

The Development of Hospitals in Tameside

The history of Tameside General Hospital reflects both the poor law and voluntary hospital traditions (Abel-Smith 1960, White 1978). The population of Ashton-under-Lyne grew rapidly during the Industrial Revolution and in 1849 a new workhouse was built to accommodate 500 people. The impetus for building a local voluntary hospital came in 1858 when Samuel Oldham left £10,000 in his will to provide care for ill or injured persons living within three-and-a-half miles of Ashton-under-Lyne (Darnton 1877). When the infirmary opened in 1861 a house surgeon was appointed and his wife employed as Matron.

By the 1930s, after the care of the poor had been transferred to the county authorities, the former workhouse began to be used solely as a hospital. The infirmary and workhouse were amalgamated to form Ashton General Hospital after the introduction of the National Health Service in 1948 and the hospital was renamed Tameside General Hospital in 1975 after local government re-organisation.

The History of the Tameside Nursing Development Unit

Until 1987 all 'geriatric' patients admitted to Tameside General Hospital were nursed in wards that had previously been part of the workhouse. Elderly people in the Tameside area still refer to that part of the hospital as the workhouse.

The Tameside Nursing Development Unit was established on the foundation of joint appointments between education and service in the 'Geriatric Unit' in the early 1980s. Kate Wilkinson, Director of Nurse Education at the time, explained the choice of clinical area by the School of Nursing in blunt terms:

I'll tell you why we chose the Care of the Elderly, it was so bad you couldn't get any lower. So if it didn't work there was nothing lost.

Mike Johnson, Divisional Nursing Officer, assessed the wards when he came to Tameside:

You name it, the Unit was deficient in every area, there was no area where I could honestly say, 'We've got it right'.

Kate Wilkinson recalled saying to Steve Wright, before he took up a joint appointment:

What I want you to do is to go out there and sort that Unit, that area out for me. We've got to help the nurses understand there is a different way of doing this, right, to show them a different vision.

By 1984–85, the additional educational support that student nurses received on the wards from the joint appointees encouraged them to apply for posts in the unit when they qualified. Reid (1985) and Fretwell (1985) reported similar benefits for students of increased teaching on the ward. The Unit was able to develop further when three new acute wards opened in 1987, so that it was possible both to improve staffing levels and reduce the number of beds in the old wards. The Care of the Elderly Unit became a Nursing Development Unit at that stage. Steve Wright recalled:

In my head was this idea of the NDU, for example as saying 'You know, we've done it now, we've cracked it, these four or five wards are on their way, there's a new unit opening, here's a great opportunity, now let's give it a formal name, let's tell everybody in the Health Authority'.

Within the NDU development opportunities were made available to all nursing staff, trained and untrained. Nurses were valued more and therefore in a better position to provide individualised care for their patients.

Social Context of the Study

The main industries in Tameside, which lies to the east of Manchester, were textiles, particularly cotton, and engineering until the recession in the early 1980s. In the cotton mills certain jobs were done by women, so there is a strong tradition in the area of women's employment (Liddington and Norris 1978). The communities that make up the towns in Tameside are stable, different generations of the same family tend to live near each other and family networks are very strong. Most of the nursing staff in this study come from the locality and nearly all of the qualified nurses did their nurse training at Tameside General Hospital. For women living in Tameside who wish to work locally, nursing offers one of the few opportunities in the area for professional training and subsequent professional status and income. Other 'women's jobs' in the area do not tend to offer similar career paths. Consequently, rapid staff turnover and problems in retaining nursing staff have not been major issues in the Care of the Elderly Unit.

The Nurses' Stories

Choice of Nursing as an Occupation

Only one question was asked in all the interviews, and this concerned why informants had chosen nursing as a job or career. I always stated that I was not a nurse, so that nurses were able to explain to me, as a lay person, an experience that they knew I had not been through myself.

This group of nurses took a variety of paths into nursing, with only a small number of them entering nursing at the age of 18, unlike the student nurses in a teaching hospital described by Smith (1992). Some of the participants in my study who started nurse training at 18 had relatives with nursing experience:

My mum . . . she'd done her training but then she went back to secretarial work cos of the hours at the time.

Financial constraints prevented other women, who had always wanted to be nurses, from training until later in their lives. One nurse commented:

When I sort of left school you had a job in the mill and that is where you went.

Family support played an important part in enabling women with children to start nursing:

Well I came into nursing when I was 30 years of age. I have three children, I had them quite young so they were sort of growing up. My youngest son had just started school at five and my mother had retired early.

A few nurses commented that when they had applied to do their training they were steered towards enrolled nurse training. One recalled:

Now at that time I didn't know the difference between registered nursing and enrolled nursing and I came for the interview and I was offered enrolled nursing and . . . I was told that due to my children's age they thought that 'Registered nursing would be too academically stressful for me'.

MacGuire (1980) refers to the encouragement given to women with children to apply for enrolled nurse training to widen the pool of potential recruits in order to reduce the perennial shortage of nurses. One nurse told me why she subsequently converted to RGN:

> It was a bit before I was 40, it was still 20 years I'd got to work you know, and I felt that enrolled nursing didn't give me the freedom I wanted.

Although most of the auxiliaries had family responsibilities, they were not permitted to intrude into their work. One person described her interview for an NA post:

> It was explained very clearly to me that if I was to ring up and say that the children were poorly that I would be dismissed instantly.

One nurse talked about her family and not wanting to take on more than she could cope with:

> I'm very close to my kids and I want to be there whenever they need me. They come first and I think if you're going to go up the ladder you've got to really – be able to put your job first quite a few times.

Nurses working nights talked about their husbands' participation in childcare. One of them said:

> When I was at work, he was at home. So it wasn't a problem at all. So they were never left, you know, on their own. There was . . . one of us there all the time for them.

Another nurse, who works nights, talked about the pressure of combining full-time work with childcare:

> I mean these girls that work on days with new babies . . . most have them have got to drive a baby to a childminder. The only other alternative I can think of is that all their husbands must work nine 'til five, that's the only way I could possibly have done, come back full-time on days.

Nurses without family responsibilities recognised the difference that this made in relation to work. One nurse who was talking about working overtime said:

> I don't get tired, me, but I haven't got a family to look after you see. I suppose if I had a family to look after it would be different.

One RGN, looking back on her nursing career, commented on the changes she had observed in nurses' orientation to work:

Nurses today have a lot of commitments, private commitments as well as work commitments. I think in those days, when you came into nursing, you just had your nursing commitments.

The nurses she came across at the beginning of her career would have been single women who devoted themselves to the job (Davies and Rosser 1986, 42).

The nurses in this study took a range of paths into nursing and made a long-term commitment to nursing as a job or career. Family responsibilities affected decisions about whether to undertake further training or work during the day rather than at night. Many of these women are now nursing at a different level, such as enrolled nurses who converted to RGN and auxiliaries who became enrolled nurses.

Going to Work on Care of the Elderly

In nursing, care of the elderly suffers from low status and there is a lingering attitude that elderly patients only require 'basic nursing care' (Redfern 1986, 389). An enrolled nurse who had been working as an auxiliary said:

> I never realised until I went into training, you only went into geriatrics if you couldn't get a job anywhere else, it was as simple as that.

One RGN, who had planned while training to work with children, obtained a staff nurse post on Care of the Elderly and just after starting work there received a phone call:

> The nursing officer on paediatrics rang me up and said 'What are you doing in that dead hole? You know I've got a job for you here if you want it. Your career is wasted on Care of the Elderly'.

One nurse explained why she had wanted to work on 'geriatrics':

> It was a part of – part of the hospital where it seemed you got the smaller slice of the cake for everything – erm – and we're all going to end up that age one day and I was horrified that my mother could end up there, or I could end up there.

One nurse suggested that Care of the Elderly is now seen in a more positive light, at least by the nurses who work there:

> I think the people who work on the Unit now, work on the Unit cos they want to work on the Unit, and not because they were sent there, which is what happened in the past.

Patient Care

The care of elderly patients has changed away from task-orientated care over the last ten years. Nurses think more carefully about their approach to patients because they can no longer rely on routine (Baker 1983). Towards the end of this study I realised that when nurses talked about their earlier years working on the Unit, they tended to focus on the routine and their relationships with other ward staff, but when they described the work that they do now, they talked a great deal about patients, who have become central to their work.

Attitudes to Elderly Patients

Elderly people in Western societies are perceived as having low status because they are no longer in employment and many elderly people, especially women, live in poverty (Groves 1987, 199, Arber and Ginn 1991, 79). One nurse commented on how assumptions made about elderly people can be incorrect:

> They must think that if they see a little lady with grey hair sat there, very quiet, that she's gone, her mind's gone, and they've got a lot to learn I'll tell you. If they took the time and the effort – erm – to involve the patient in their care and find out what they want . . . and what they are capable of doing, you see some smashing results, the end . . . results are great, you know.

Another nurse talked, in relation to a particular patient, about age not being the main aspect of someone's personality:

> You can get somebody, they're old at 50 you know, they've always been old and you get somebody who is quite youthful at 80 or 90. Like this lady at 100 she said to me, 'I know it sounds silly', she said, 'but in here [she pointed at her head] I only feel 50 but I can't do the same as I did at 50'. She said, 'I don't really feel any different'. So it's a state of mind isn't it really, age?

Other nurses talked about how the current generation of elderly people have experienced two world wars, and working lives that are very different from those of younger people. One nursing auxiliary said:

> I love listening to old people, I like listening to, you know, what they used to do when they were younger in their life . . . and how many children did they have and how could they err afford it, and where did they go to have their babies, if they had them at home and all that.

The way that the positive attitudes towards elderly people expressed by nurses in this study differ from those found in other studies of nursing suggests that a shift away from traditional nursing culture has taken place.

Talking to Patients

A nurse in the Day Hospital described how she approached anxious patients:

> We have had them come in here and they've been so uptight you know, really tense, and I've sat down with them and I've said, 'There's something worrying you'. 'I'll be alright, I'll be alright' and gradually just by sitting there and touching them it will all come out.

Nurses felt that they were now able to communicate more effectively with patients. One nursing auxiliary said:

> You can enjoy it now, you can be a human being with them, you can, if they're feeling sad you can be sad with them. You don't have to have this big front up like you used to, stand back from them emotions and crying you know, if somebody'd died, get them [the relatives] out of the way quick. You don't have to do that any more, you can stay with them, and you can put your arm around them you know, you can be with them.

These two nurses provided examples from their own experience of the skill that Benner (1984) describes as 'presencing', which emphasises the importance of touch and person-to-person contact between patient and nurse and the need for nurses to allow patients to express their feelings.

Another nursing auxiliary said that female patients talked to nurses about how they felt about their lives:

> You get a lot of them reliving what they should have done . . . and what they did do, and they're sorry at the way their life's gone, you know what they should have done, looked after themselves more, and not done so much for the family.

However, if nurses are expected to give more of themselves by becoming more involved with patients, they may find that they are unable to respond appropriately to all patients. One nurse described how nurses negotiated between themselves who would care for individual patients:

> You've got to have a mixture of people, there's no point us all having the same things . . . You can go on a ward and the first patient you look at, you think, 'God, I hate him.' And even though you're very polite, the fact that you're polite tells the patient there's something wrong – erm – so, but the next staff that comes in thinks they're wonderful, whereas the one

across the way they can think, 'Oh I'm not going to that bed, you go'. And you can think, 'Well why? She's wonderful'.

One RGN found that not having enough time to talk to patients caused her concern:

I mean to me that's more important, talking to them, than anything else . . . You sometimes think, Oh God, I haven't even said, all I've said is 'Hiya' to one person and I thought that's really bad. You think they've sat there all day with nothing to do and they're just looking round at everyone running round and nobody speaks to them, and it really does wind me up sometimes.

Talking to patients enables nurses to give them information about their illness and find out how much they understand about why they have been in hospital. One RGN said:

You'll tell them one little bit one day, then you'll tell them a bit more the next day. I mean some patients you can [tell] they don't want to know so obviously we just discuss it with the relatives, or we try to tell them the basics before they go home so they know why, or what's happened to them.

Nurses on the Care of the Elderly Unit now see talking to patients as an integral part of their work. Talking to patients can show that they are valued as people, provide reassurance, emotional support, companionship and information. The information that nurses acquire through talking to patients enables them to respond to patients' needs on a more individual basis.

Meeting Patients' Needs

If elderly people are treated as individuals, their needs are more likely to be met. One RGN commented:

Ultimately, no matter what, their needs are their needs and they're very important to them when they're poorly. No matter how trivial they seem to us.

Two nurses talked about the changes that have taken place in relation to the information that patients have access to:

N1   At one time patients weren't allowed to sort of know what they were being, what their treatment [was] and everything, now they can ask and get told, they're not kept in the dark the same are they?

N2   No, at one time . . .

N1   The treatment, the nursing processes are kept at the bedside so they can read them if they want.

N2   At one time it was a case of you know, like say give somebody a tablet, they'd say, 'What's this?' and it were a case of like, 'Doesn't matter, you take it'. Well it's not like that now, is it? You know, you can say, you might say, 'Do you want any pain-killers?' Whereas you just used to give them [to patients] didn't you?

One nurse who works nights talked about how she assessed patients by observing them without going from bed to bed in a routine way:

Most nurses do this routine in as much as we go, we'll go into a bay and we'll stand there and we'll say, 'Are you alright, gents? Do you want them pillows doing?' . . . And then you're assessing the others whilst you're in there and they, you can see the one that erm needs their bed doing so you go and then you do their bed and then the other one in the meantime has got up and gone and you'll say, 'Are you walking to the toilet all night or do you want a bottle?' You're not interested whether he walks or not, you know, it's just a point of conversation. If he turns round and answers you briskly, well you know he's OK, if he turns round slowly you can tell by this.

One RGN talked about mobilising patients and how nurses' attitudes have changed:

I think probably one of the factors that held them [nurses] back was the risk element. They weren't prepared to actually acknowledge that the patients had the right to take that risk, to get up and walk you know. Whereas now we would say, 'Well okay if you want to walk, I'll walk with you', then they would say, 'No, you can't walk because you'll fall', instead of allowing them the right to take that risk. And I think in nursing the elderly there is always going to be an element of risk, but you can't take away their independence simply because you are a nurse.

One aspect of meeting the needs of patients which causes difficulties for nurses is the differences between patients in their levels of expectations and assertiveness. Nurses were aware that if they responded to all the requests of the articulate patients, the needs of other patients might not be met. One nursing auxiliary working on a rehabilitation ward said:

You get about five on a ward and them will have all the attention and you get all these quiet ones who'll just sit back and never speak all day . . . And you can bet if you were talking to this lonely little lady whatever, one of the chatty ones would shout you for something else.

In a later interview I asked one RGN how she dealt with competing demands from patients:

N   Oh I just try to share myself out between everybody, give myself, give them all the same.

MB   Right, so if you get one persistent person . . .

N   I just tell him I've got to go and see to some others. Unless genuinely if they're very ill and they're shouting because they want something . . . But if I know that they're just shouting because they want all the attention, I'll just explain to them that I've got to give my time to the others . . . If I know someone is quiet, I won't just, you know, not bother with them, I always go and say something to them.

Though nurses wish to provide individualised care for patients, meeting the needs of patients is not always straightforward. The quotations above illustrate some of the difficulties encountered by nurses in this study, and in some cases the ways in which they try to overcome them.

What Gave Them Satisfaction?

Job satisfaction is an issue that brings together themes that have been explored above, such as being a nurse and different aspects of caring for elderly patients. Nurses expressed their attitudes towards their jobs in different ways.

Standards of Patient Care

One nursing auxiliary referred back to how depressing some aspects of the work had been:

They were terrible, the pressure sores then – and they didn't have the treatments for pressure, you know that they have now, and they've all these new beds and mattresses which is a big improvement. They take care they don't get any [pressure sores]. There were some awful sights on there, very depressing.

Another nursing auxiliary commented:

I think it's got better, much nicer, much better atmosphere, patients and staff have a much better relationship. They used to be frightened . . . of asking for anything, and I don't know why, because I always feel that I'm approachable, you know I mean I don't like to feel that anybody couldn't ask me for something, that'd be awful.

Another nurse referred to the changes that have improved the quality of life for patients:

Everything has sort of done an about change now and it's patient choice and that is individual care and that's brilliant really now . . . All the regimentation has gone through the window which is good really. I wouldn't mind being a patient sometimes.

Although nurses valued the changes that had taken place, some commented on the increased demands made on them. One RGN said:

We're having to do all these new things with the same amount of staff as we had when we weren't doing them and like it's just a constant pressure to have to do all these things and we never get any time to learn how to do them . . . We've got to do it all in our own time . . . but sometimes when you're at home and you've been dead busy you don't feel like doing it all.

Other nurses said that they sometimes felt that changes were introduced for the sake of change, which meant that it was difficult to take on new ideas and try to implement them properly.

Working as a Team

Nurses talked about working as part of a team. One nursing auxiliary referred to the changing role of sisters:

Well sisters pull their weight a lot now, you know, they're very good. On our side, they all, they don't only sit in the office all the day, they muck in on the wards, so they see what's going on you know, that's changed a lot.

Nurses who worked on night duty talked about their relationships with other nurses. One auxiliary said:

There's not very many of us and you are more dependent on each other, aren't you. I think we work better as a team than day time and mostly people on nights are not ladder climbers either.

Some informants took the view that nurses did not help each other as much as they had in the past. One EN said:

No one seems to – I can't say they don't care, but no one seems to notice whether another ward is particular busy, they all sort of centre round their own ward and that's it.

Personal Satisfaction

Nurses talked about the personal satisfaction that they derive from their work. A nursing auxiliary commented:

It's strange, I think once you've been in it with the elderly, there's something that draws you all the time. I'm happy while I'm at work you know and I feel I've done something good when I get home. Better than working in a factory, it's just the routine in there, but this is something different every day. I mean you see a lot of sadness of course you know, but you get a lot of pleasure. My husband still doesn't understand why I ever came into this job.

Another nursing auxiliary talked about how her job had changed:

I feel that I'm a carer now, where before I weren't nursing, it were just a routine, like a machine really. You didn't have time to talk to patients, you just went to them, washed them, fed them and that was it. But now you can sit and talk.

One RGN said:

I've said many a time I can go home and go to bed and I've done a good night's work . . . If I can do that I'm OK. I said the day I go home and I know I haven't, that's the day to chuck it in and call it a day – I don't know, I just like nursing, that's all.

Commitment to their job affects nurses' quality of life outside their work. One RGN commented:

I said I used to have so much outside interests, I don't have nothing, nothing at all, only work . . . You can be a very boring person, I think, if work's everything, cos when you go out for a drink you're talking about work whereas before I could talk about a lot of things.

Nurses also talked about their preference for nursing different types of patient. One RGN commented:

It's very rewarding . . . to see somebody that's had a stroke and you've rehabilitated them to the point where they are able to go home . . . Maybe they was incontinent and you've been able to help them within a pattern, they're not just left to be incontinent and to dribble and put in a long-stay type of care, you're giving them some sort of dignity.

Other nurses talked about how they preferred the faster pace on acute wards. One nurse said:

You might be on seven days before your days off, and you think, oh seven days, long time, but it flies by and it's always a bit of variety every day, different patients you've got or what's happening on the ward. And the unexpected always happens, you know, so it keeps you going.

Nurses talked about their work, and expressed their satisfaction with nursing or the lack of it in different ways, which reflect the choices, experiences and influences that have affected participants in this study since their entry into nursing.

Discussion and Conclusions

From his study of the difference between the idealised picture of nurses and the experience of women who were recruited to nurse in provincial hospitals during the late nineteenth century and early twentieth century, Maggs (1980, 38) concludes:

> Altogether the nurse recruit was much more like her fellow women worker than we might have gathered from the nursing histories, and that discovering her involves looking beyond nursing itself and towards the study of women in British society.

The gap between media portrayal and reality probably still exists and the way that nursing is portrayed by nurse leaders is closely linked to the quest for professional status and recognition for nursing (Witz 1990). There are still major differences between the educational qualifications required for nurse training by metropolitan teaching hospitals and provincial general hospitals. As research funding tends to be concentrated in metropolitan hospitals, more is known about nurses who work there than in local general hospitals. This study, which presents a 'view from below' (Harraway 1988), shows paths into nursing that differed from the traditional entry point of 18 for school leavers, and constraints on the occupational choices of nursing staff because of their family responsibilities.

These barriers made it difficult for women in this study to enter nursing and with the unpromising environment of a former workhouse in which to care for patients and the low status of elderly care in nursing, high levels of job satisfaction might not have been expected. However, the way that nurses described the rewarding nature of their work in this chapter is supported by further evidence. The motivation to provide good quality patient care that had emerged in the interviews was also reflected in the survey of NDU staff that I conducted early in 1992 (Black 1993a). Though nurses in my survey expressed dissatisfaction with some aspects of their working conditions, particularly staff shortages, their morale was higher than that found by Waite and Hutt (1987) and Seccombe and Ball (1992) in their surveys of Royal College of Nursing (RCN) members.

Nurses showed very high levels of satisfaction (over 90 per cent) with the level of responsibilities they had dealt with, and the standard of physical care that they had provided in the previous week in the survey I carried out. Three-quarters of nursing staff (70 out of 93) were satisfied with the level of psychological/social aspects of care that they had provided. Further comparisons were made between the responses of Tameside NDU nurses and RCN members in Waite and Hutt's survey to the same questions about certain features of working life relating to patient care, professional autonomy and working conditions. Tameside NDU nurses were more likely to perceive that they could offer high-quality nursing care to their patients than nurses in the national RCN sample, although nurses in the RCN survey worked in a range of clinical settings, including the more prestigious high-technology specialities.

This study set out to explore the perceptions of nurses who had been caught up in the process of change. The picture of nursing elderly patients portrayed in this chapter is far less depressing than that found in other studies (Wells 1980, Baker 1983, Smith 1992), both in the positive attitudes to elderly patients and in nurses' confidence in their ability to provide good patient care. Changes designed to improve the way that patients were cared for in the Care of the Elderly Unit at Tameside General Hospital have made an impact on nursing practice. The nurses in this study talk in a thoughtful, reflective way about how they care for their patients, which shows that they have moved beyond what Fretwell (1985, 125) describes as a:

'veneer of change' through documentation, whilst leaving underlying practices untouched.

The nurses in this study did not express concerns about the undervaluing of women's work, particularly in those jobs which are not seen as highly skilled because they build on caring and domestic work within the home. They came into nursing when their domestic circumstances made this possible, because they wanted to be nurses and to care for people. Several nurses described to me the conflict between their personal values and the way that they were expected to work when they started to work in the Unit (Black 1993b). The changes that took place increased nurses' self-esteem and they overcame the stigma of elderly care, nursing mainly elderly women, discovering its rewards through the closer relationships with patients that came about as a result of the professional support they received.

Herzberg, Mausner and Snyderman (1959, 114) in their study of *The Motivation to Work* distinguish between conditions of work and 'the need to develop in one's occupation as a source of personal growth'. Working in a different way made nurses in this study feel better about themselves and see the work they do as important. They were also more conscious of their nursing identity, and their role as patients' advocate that enabled them to become more assertive with doctors (Black 1993a). This study shows that change which benefits both nurses and patients can be brought about, despite resource constraints, if there is a shared commitment at all levels within the organisation and a network of support for nursing staff.

Note

The study on which this chapter was based was funded by the Department of Health and administered by the King's Fund Centre. The views expressed are mine and do not necessarily reflect those of the sponsors of the research.

References

Abel-Smith B (1960) *A History of the Nursing Profession*. London: Heinemann.

Arber S and Ginn J (1991) *Gender and Later Life*. London: Sage Publications.

Baker D E (1983) Care in the geriatric ward: an account of two styles of nursing. In Wilson-Barnett J (ed.) *Nursing Research: Ten Studies in Patient Care*. Chichester: John Wiley and Sons.

Benner P (1984) *From Novice to Expert*. Menlo Park, California: Addison Wesley.

Black M (1993a) *The Growth of Tameside Nursing Development Unit: An Exploration of Perceived Changes in Nursing Practice over a Ten Year Period*. London: King's Fund Centre.

Black M (1993b) *A Different Vision: Nurses' Perceptions of Change in an Elderly Care Nursing Development Unit*. MSc thesis, Department of Nursing, University of Manchester.

Cockburn C (1991) *In the Way of Women: Men's Resistance to Sex Equality in Organisations*. Basingstoke: Macmillan Education.

Darnton H T (1877) *An Historical Sketch of the Origin of the District Infirmary Ashton-under-Lyne*. Ashton-under-Lyne: Griffin and Sheard.

Davies C and Rosser J (1986) *Processes of Discrimination: A Report on a Study of Women Working in the NHS*. London: DHSS.

Dex S (ed.) (1991) *Life and Work History Analyses: Qualitative and Quantitative Developments*. Sociological Review Monograph 37. London: Routledge.

Fretwell J E (1985) *Freedom to Change: The Creation of a Ward Learning Environment*. London: Royal College of Nursing.

Gamarnikow E (1978) Sexual division of labour: the case of nursing. In Kuhn A and Wolpe A M (eds) *Feminism and Materialism*. London: Routledge and Kegan Paul.

Groves D (1987) Occupational pension provision and women's poverty in old age. In Glendinning C and Millar J (eds). *Women and Poverty in Britain*. Brighton: Wheatsheaf Books.

Harraway D (1988) Situated knowledges: the science question in feminism and the privilege of partial perspective. *Feminist Studies*, **14**, 3, 575–599.

Herzberg F, Mausner B and Snyderman B B (1959) *The Motivation to Work*. New York: John Wiley and Sons.

Hochschild A R (1983) *The Managed Heart*. Berkeley: University of California Press.

James N (1989) Emotional labour: skill and work in the social regulation of feelings. *Sociological Review*, **37**, 1, 15–42.

Joshi H (1985) Motherhood and employment: change and continuity in post-war Britain. In British Society for Population Studies, *Measuring Socio-demographic Change*, Occasional paper 34. London: Office of Population Censuses and Surveys.

Liddington J and Norris J (1978) *One Hand Tied Behind Us: The Rise of the Women's Suffrage Movement*. London: Virago.

MacGuire J (1980) Nursing: None is held in higher esteem. Occupational control and the position of women in nursing. In Silverstone R and Ward A (eds) *Careers of Professional Women*. London: Croom Helm.

Maggs C (1980) Nurse recruitment to four provincial hospitals 1881–1991. In Davies C (ed.) *Rewriting Nursing History*. London: Croom Helm.

Redfern S (1986) The elderly patient. In Redfern S (ed.) *Nursing Elderly People*. Edinburgh: Churchill Livingstone.

Reid N G (1985) *Wards in Chancery? Nurse Training in the Clinical Area*. London: Royal College of Nursing.

Salvage J (1992) The new nursing: empowering patients or empowering nurses? In Robinson J, Gray A and Elkan R (eds) *Policy Issues in Nursing*. Buckingham: Open University Press.

Seccombe I and Ball J (1992) *Motivation, Morale and Mobility: A Profile of Trained Nurses in the 1990s*. IMS Report 233. Brighton: Institute of Manpower Studies.

Smith P (1992) *The Emotional Labour of Nursing*. Basingstoke: Macmillan Education.

Waite R and Hutt R (1987) *Attitudes, Jobs and Mobility of Qualified Nurses: a report for the Royal College of Nursing*. Brighton: Institute of Manpower Studies.

Wells T J (1980) *Problems in Geriatric Nursing Care*. Edinburgh: Churchill Livingstone.

White R (1978) *Social Change and the Development of the Nursing Profession. A Study of the Poor Law Service 1848–1948*. London: Henry Kimpton.

Wilson D C (1992) *A Strategy of Change: Concepts and Controversies in the Management of Change*. London: Routledge.

Witz A (1990) Patriarchy and professions: the gendered politics of occupational closure. *Sociology*, **24**, 4, 675–690.

Index